中国传统文化「走出去」丛书之二
Chinese Traditional Culture "Going Out" Series II

林记明 孙佐枫 丛书主编

十二段锦（中英双语）
Shi'erduanjin
(Chinese-English)

孙佐枫 著
林记明 译

河北出版传媒集团
河北人民出版社
石家庄

图书在版编目（CIP）数据

十二段锦 / 孙佐枫著；林记明译. -- 石家庄：河北人民出版社，2023.11
（中国传统文化"走出去"丛书. 之二）
ISBN 978-7-202-16565-2

Ⅰ. ①十… Ⅱ. ①孙… ②林… Ⅲ. ①气功－健身运动－基本知识 Ⅳ. ①R214

中国国家版本馆CIP数据核字(2023)第237563号

丛 书 名	中国传统文化"走出去"丛书之二
	ZHONGGUO CHUANTONG WENHUA ZOUCHUQU CONGSHU ZHIER
丛书主编	林记明　孙佐枫
书　　名	十二段锦
	SHIERDUANJIN
著　　者	孙佐枫
译　　者	林记明
总 策 划	王斌贤
策划编辑	路殿国　李成轩
责任编辑	付　聪
美术编辑	王　婧
责任校对	余尚敏
摄　　影	蔡欣然
出版发行	河北出版传媒集团　河北人民出版社
	（石家庄市友谊北大街330号）
印　　刷	河北新华第一印刷有限责任公司
开　　本	787毫米×1092毫米　1/16
印　　张	8
字　　数	106 000
版　　次	2023年11月第1版　2023年11月第1次印刷
书　　号	ISBN 978-7-202-16565-2
定　　价	29.00元

版权所有　翻印必究

<<< 前言
Foreword

十二段锦属古代导引术，由十二段动作组成。用"锦"字来命名，表示作为一套完整的坐式导引功法，犹如一幅精美华贵、连绵不断的画卷。十二段锦之名称最早出现在清代乾隆年间徐文弼编辑的《寿世传真》一书，其功法内容则来源于"钟离八段锦法"。"钟离八段锦法"出自明朝《正统道藏》第122至131册中的《修真十书》。据李远国编著《中国道教气功养生大全》记载，《修真十书》"主要收集了隋唐两宋时期几十种重要的气功和内丹著作"。

Shi'erduanjin is a Chinese ancient *Daoyin* exercise composed of twelve postures. Named with the Chinese character " 锦 (jin)", it represents a complete set of sitting *Daoyin* movements, just like an exquisite, magnificent and continuous painting scroll. The name of Shi'erduanjin first appeared in the book *Transmission of Truth in the Longevity World* edited by Xu Wenbi during the Qianlong period of the Qing Dynasty. The content of its exercise originated from the "Zhongli Baduanjin" found in *Ten books on Cultivating Perfection* in Volumes 122 to 131 of the *Orthodox Daoist Canon* in the Ming Dynasty. According to *The Complete Book of Daoist Qigong Health Preservation in China* compiled by Li Yuanguo, the *Ten Books on Cultivating Perfection* mainly collected dozens of important *Qigong* and internal alchemy works during the Sui, Tang and Song dynasties.

《修真十书·钟离八段锦法》的歌诀及阐释为：闭目冥心坐，握固静思神。叩齿三十六，两手抱昆仑。左右鸣天鼓，二十四度闻。微摆撼天柱，赤龙搅水浑。漱津三十六，神水满口匀。一口分三咽，龙行虎自奔。闭气搓手热，背摩后精门。尽此一口气，想火烧脐轮。左右辘轳转，两脚放舒伸。叉手双虚托，低头攀足频。以候逆水上，再漱再吞津。如此三度毕，神水九次吞。咽下汨汨响，百脉自调匀。河车搬运讫，发火遍烧身。邪魔不敢近，梦寐不能昏。寒暑不能入，灾病不能迍。子后午前作，造化合乾坤。循环次第转，八卦是良因。

The Song of "Zhongli Baduanjin" reads: Sit in meditation with eyes closed, hands clenched. Click teeth thirty-six times, hold *Kunlun* in both hands. Sound celestial drums twenty-four times. Slightly shake the heavenly column, stir the tongue inside the mouth. Gargle with saliva thirty-six times until your mouth is full of it. Swallow it in three gulps, feeling dragon and tiger running within you. While holding breath, rub your hands warm and massage essence gates in the lower back. While breathing out, imagine fire burning at the navel ring. Rotate your left or right arm like windlass, stretch out your legs. Raise your interlocked hands up, bend down to touch the toes. Once saliva fills your mouth, gargle thirty-three times again and swallow it in three gulps, three rounds in all. Swallow with a gurgling sound to unblock meridians. Finish with the transportation of *Qi*, feeling the heat spreading throughout your body. Since demons dare not approach, you won't suffer insomnia. Cold and heat cannot penetrate, disasters and diseases cannot befall. Perform this exercise after midnight and before noon, aligning with the harmony of heaven and earth. The cycle repeats itself with the Eight Trigrams as the cause.

十二段锦又称"坐式八段锦"。是中国古代养生方法的杰出代表。受到明、清众多医学家、养生家的大力推崇。它吸收了中国传统文化的精华，将医疗、运动、养生有机地结合起来，以提高生命质量、完善生命状态为基本目标，提倡通过自我的运动、锻炼，来达到身、心的和谐统一。十二段锦的养生思想，系统反映了中国传统养生道法自然、内外兼修的锻炼原则。尤其是对于放松身心有良好作用。本书中英文对照，从功法操作、学练要领、功理功用和适宜症状等方面进行通俗易懂的论述。

Shi'erduanjin, also known as "Sitting Baduanjin", is an outstanding representative of ancient Chinese health-preserving exercises. It was highly praised by many medical and health experts during the Ming and Qing dynasties. It absorbs the essence of traditional Chinese culture, integrating medical treatment, sport, and health preservation, with the goal of enhancing the quality of life and attaining a state of well-being. It advocates a harmonious unity between body and mind through self-exercise and training. The philosophy of Shi'erduanjin systematically reflects the training principles of traditional Chinese health preservation, which emphasize following nature with internal and external cultivation. It is particularly effective for relaxing the body and mind. This book in Chinese and English contains instructions, key points, functions and effects, and indications, which are easy to understand.

全套动作简单易学易练。适合不同年龄的人进行锻炼，长期坚持可有效地增进身体健康，达到防病强身的作用。非常适宜在中外健身人群中普及推广。在倡导文化自信，建设文化强国和健康中国的时代背景下，对中国传统文化的国际传播具有文化和健身方面的重要价值。

The entire set of postures is easy to learn and practice for people of different ages, and long-term practice can effectively improve physical health and prevent diseases. Therefore, it is very suitable for Chinese and foreign fitness enthusiasts. In the context of advocating cultural confidence and building a strong cultural and healthy China, this book is of great cultural and health value to the international dissemination of traditional Chinese culture.

<<< 目录
Contents

预备势 / 001
Preparation / 001

第一式　冥心握固 / 005
Posture 1　Calm Mind and Clench Hands / 005

第二式　叩齿鸣鼓 / 008
Posture 2　Click Teeth and Sound Drums / 008

第三式　微撼天柱 / 015
Posture 3　Slightly Shake Heavenly Column / 015

第四式　掌抱昆仑 / 026
Posture 4　Hold *Kunlun* in Hands / 026

第五式　摇转辘轳 / 037
Posture 5　Rotate Arms like Windlass / 037

第六式　托天按顶 / 053
Posture 6　Hold Up Heaven and Press Crown / 053

第七式　俯身攀足 / 062
Posture 7　Bend to Touch Feet / 062

第八式　背摩精门 / 073
Posture 8　Massage Essence Gates / 073

第九式　前抚脘腹 / 080
Posture 9　Caress Upper and Lower Abdomen / 080

第十式　温煦脐轮 / 092
Posture 10　Warm Navel Ring / 092

第十一式　摇身晃海 / 096
Posture 11　Rotate Upper Body / 096

第十二式　鼓漱吞津 / 102
Posture 12　Gargle and Swallow / 102

收势 / 110
Closing / 110

十二段锦的呼吸要求 / 116
Breathing Requirements / 116

学习建议 / 118
Learning Tips / 118

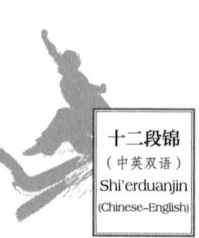

预备势

Preparation

一、功法操作
I. Instructions

动作一：两脚并拢，脚尖向前，两腿自然站立；两肩放松，两臂自然垂于体侧，身体中正安舒；目视前方。（图1）

Movement 1: Stand naturally with feet together, toes pointing forward, shoulders relaxed, arms naturally hanging at the sides of your body. Keep your body centered and comfortable. Eyes look ahead. (Figure 1)

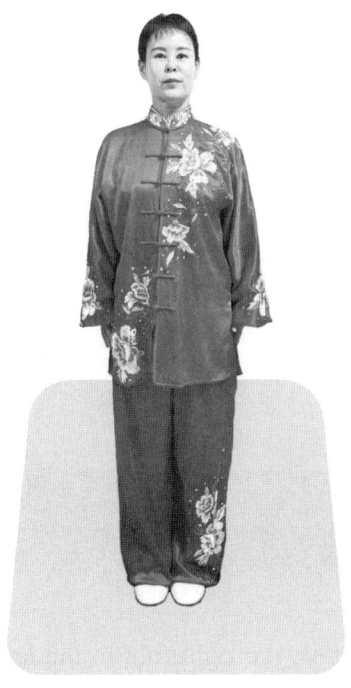

图 1/Figure 1

动作二：右膝微屈，左脚向后撤步（约肩宽的一半），前脚掌点地；目视前方。（图2）

Movement 2: Bend your right knee slightly and take a step back with your left foot (about half the width of your shoulder), landing on the ball of your foot. Eyes look ahead. (Figure 2)

动作三：两腿屈膝下蹲，两手五指撑地，稍宽于肩，两肘微屈，上体稍前倾；目视前下方。（图3）

Movement 3: Squat down with both knees bent and place both hands on the ground with the fingers spread slightly wider than your shoulders, elbows slightly bent, your upper body slightly tilted forward. Eyes look down to the front. (Figure 3)

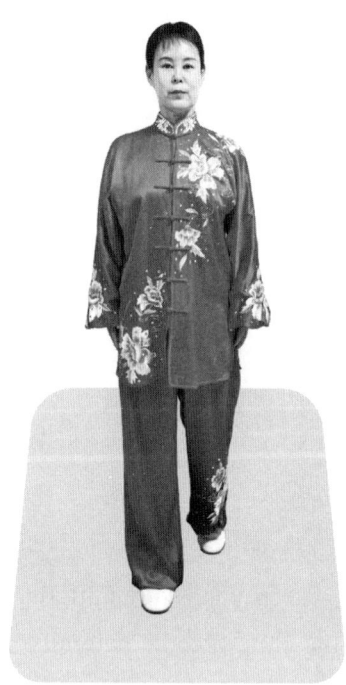
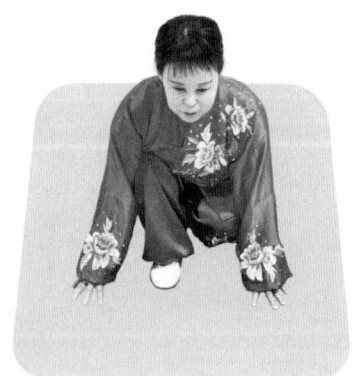

图2/Figure 2　　　　　　图3/Figure 3

动作四：右脚左移至左小腿左侧下方，脚外侧着地；目视前下方。（图4）

Movement 4: Move the right foot to the left and place it under the left calf, with the outer edge of the foot touching the ground. Eyes

look down to the front. (Figure 4)

动作五：上动不停，身体重心左移，正身盘坐，两掌扶于两膝内侧；目视前方。（图5）

Movement 5: Without a pause, shift the weight to the left and sit cross-legged with both palms on the inner knees. Eyes look ahead. (Figure 5)

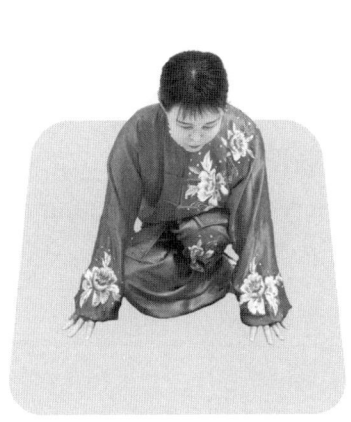
图4/Figure 4

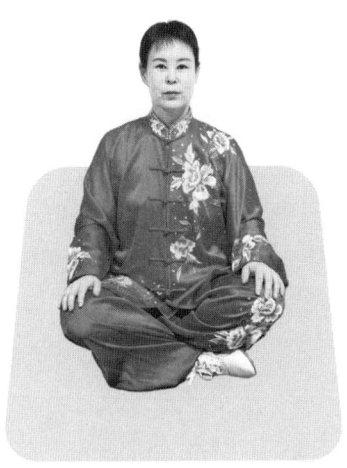
图5/Figure 5

二、学练要领
II. Key Points

1. 并步站立时，百会穴虚领，下颏微收，周身中正，唇齿合拢，自然呼吸，内心平静。

When standing with feet together, keep your body upright, pull up *Baihui* acupoint, slightly tuck in the chin, breathe naturally, and calm your mind, lips and teeth closed.

2. 习练预备势时，退步、下蹲和盘坐动作，要求速度均匀，身体平稳，正身端坐。

In Preparation, the backward step, squatting, and cross-legged sitting should be performed with even speed, your upper body stable and upright.

三、功理功用
III. Functions and Effects

本势动作可协调四肢，端正身形，调整呼吸，安定心神。

This posture can coordinate the limbs, straighten your upper body, regulate breathing and calm your mind.

四、适宜症状
IV. Indications

可缓解精神紧张、焦虑、神经衰弱等相关症状。

It can relieve mental stress, anxietys, neurasthenia and other related symptoms.

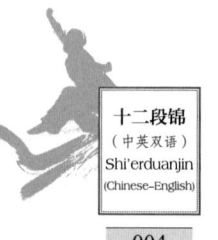

第一式　冥心握固

Posture 1　Calm Mind and Clench Hands

一、功法操作

I. Instructions

动作一：接预备势，两掌分别从两膝内侧向体侧约 45 度前伸，掌心向下；目视前下方。（图 6）

Movement 1: Continuing from the end of the Preparation, extend both palms from the inner knees to the sides of your body at about a 45-degree angle, facing down. Eyes look down to the front. (Figure 6)

动作二：上动不停，两臂外旋向斜上方举起，肘关节微屈；随之抬头，目视前上方。（图 7）

Movement 2: Without a pause, rotate both arms outward and raise them diagonally upward, elbows slightly bent. Raise your head, eyes looking up to the front. (Figure 7)

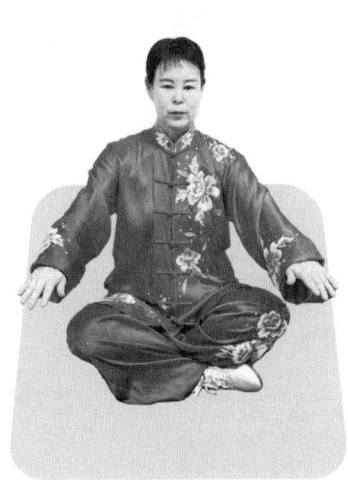
图 6/Figure 6

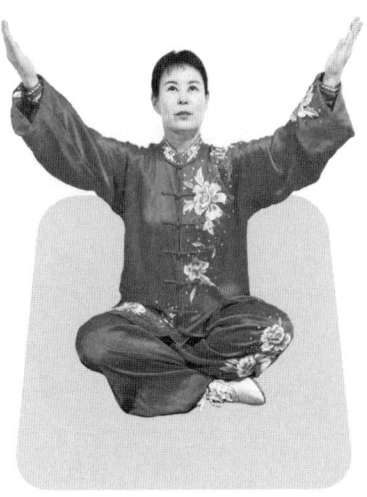
图 7/Figure 7

动作三：下颏内收，两臂内旋，两掌下落至前平举，与肩同宽，掌心向下；目视前方。（图 8）

Movement 3: Tuck in your chin. With both arms rotating inward, lower both palms to a horizontal position in front of your body, shoulder-width apart, facing down. Eyes look ahead. (Figure 8)

动作四：上动不停，两掌由身前下按，随之两手拇指抵无名指根节握固，置于两膝内侧；两眼垂帘约 30 秒钟。（图 9）（图 10 握固）

Movement 4: Without a pause, press the palms downward in front of your body. Then clench your hands with the thumb pressing against the base of the ring finger and place them on the inner knees. Close your eyes for about 30 seconds. (Figure 9) (Figure 10 clenched hand)

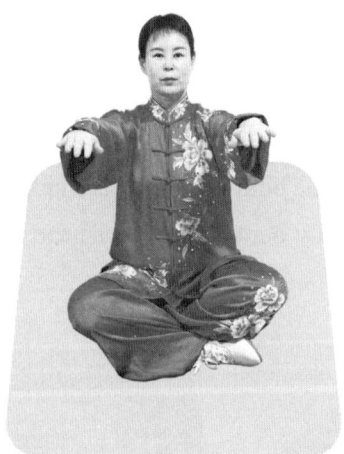
图 8/Figure 8

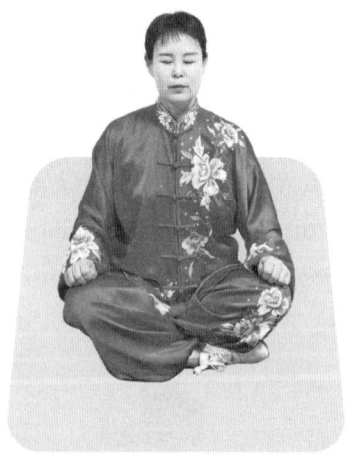
图 9/Figure 9

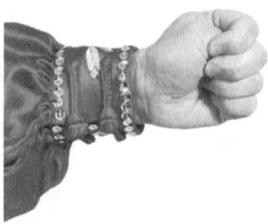
图 10 握固/Figure 10 clenched hand

二、学练要领
II. Key Points

1. 两臂上举时，舒胸展体；两掌下按时，立项竖脊，百会虚领。

When raising both arms, relax the chest and expand your upper body. When lowering both palms, straighten your neck and spine, *Baihui* acupoint gently pulled up.

2. 垂帘时，轻闭双目，排除杂念，宁心静气。

When closing your eyes gently, clear your mind of distractions and calm down.

三、功理功用
III. Functions and Effects

1. 冥心可净化大脑，颐养身心，使心气归一，启动气机。

Calming the mind can purify your brain, nourish your body, coordinate the mind and *Qi*, and activate the circulation of *Qi*.

2. 握固可以镇惊守魄，疏肝理肺。

Clenching the hands can calm the mind and protect the soul, and soothe the liver and lungs.

四、适宜症状
IV. Indications

对心悸、失眠、头昏、乏力、神经衰弱等病症有一定的防治作用。

It can help to prevent and treat symptoms such as palpitations, insomnia, dizziness, fatigue, and neurasthenia.

第二式　叩齿鸣鼓

Posture 2　Click Teeth and Sound Drums

一、功法操作

I. Instructions

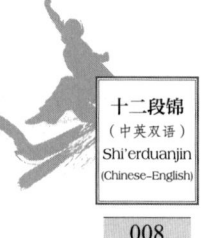

动作一：接上式，两拳变掌，收至腰间，掌心向下；目视前方。（图 11）

Movement 1: Continuing from the end of the previous posture, open your fists into palms and bring them to the waist, facing down. Eyes look ahead. (Figure 11)

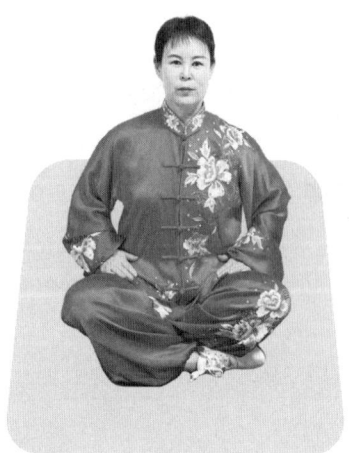

图 11/Figure 11

动作二：上动不停，两臂经腰间内旋向体侧平举，掌心向后；目视前方。（图 12）

Movement 2: Without a pause, rotate both arms inward at the waist and raise them to the sides of your body at shoulder level, palms facing back. Eyes look ahead. (Figure 12)

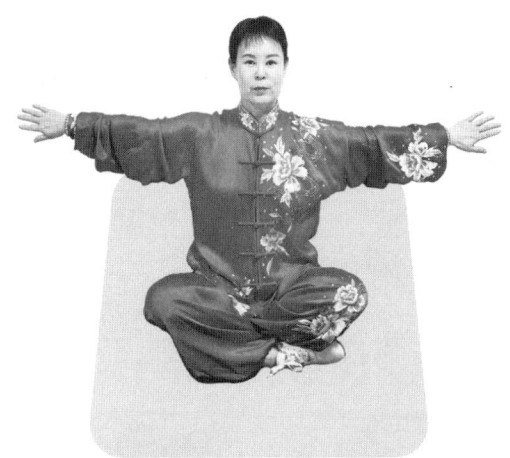

图 12/Figure 12

动作三：上动不停，两臂外旋，掌心向前；目视前方。（图13）

Movement 3: Without a pause, rotate both arms outward, palms facing forward. Eyes look ahead. (Figure 13)

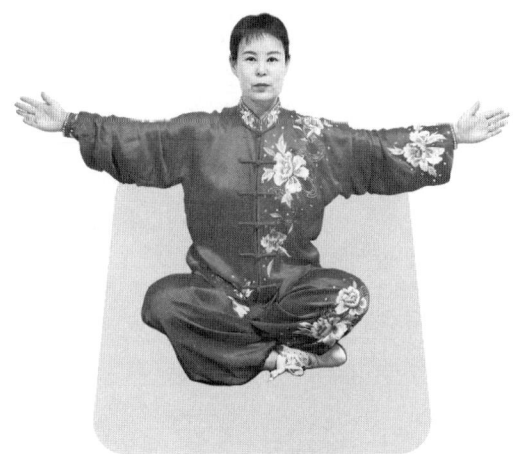

图 13/Figure 13

动作四：上动不停，两臂屈肘，两掌变通天指，中指掩实耳孔，随之叩齿 36 次；目视前下方。（图 14）（图 15 通天指）

Movement 4: Without a pause, bend the elbows and change your palms into "sky-reaching" fingers, middle fingers covering the ear holes. Then click the teeth thirty-six times. Eyes look down to the front. (Figure 14) (Figure 15 sky-reaching finger)

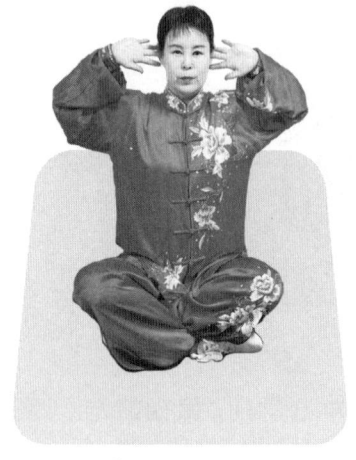
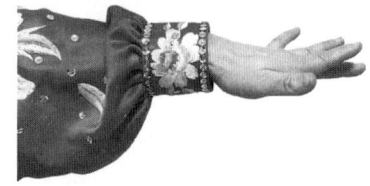

图 14/Figure 14　　　图 15 通天指/Figure 15 sky-reaching finger

动作五：两中指拔耳（拔离耳孔）；目视前下方。（图 16）

Movement 5: Pull the middle fingers away from the ear holes. Eyes look down to the front. (Figure 16)

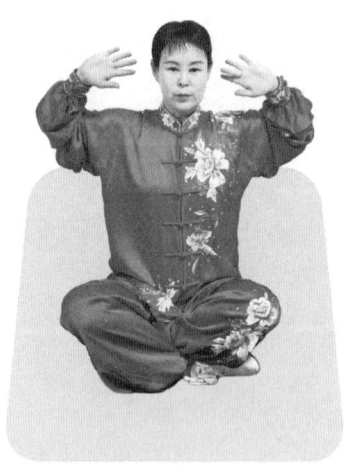

图 16/Figure 16

动作六：两手心按实耳孔，十指轻扶后脑，中指腹位于枕骨粗隆处；目视前下方。（图 17）

Movement 6: Press the ear holes with both palms, holding the back of your head lightly with the ten fingers, middle fingers on the bump of the occipital bone. Eyes look down to the front. (Figure 17)

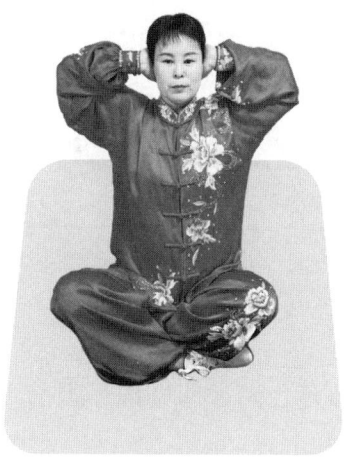

图 17/Figure 17

动作七：上动不停，两手食指分别放在两手中指上，用食指弹击后脑 24 次；目视前下方。（图 18）

Movement 7: Without a pause, place the index fingers on top of the middle fingers, and tap the back of your head twenty-four times with the index fingers. Eyes look down to the front. (Figure 18)

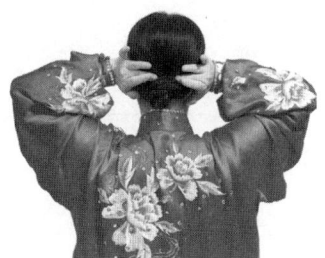

图 18/Figure 18

动作八：两手拔耳，掌心斜向前；目视前方。（图 19）

Movement 8: Remove the palms from the ears, facing diagonally forward. Eyes look ahead. (Figure 19)

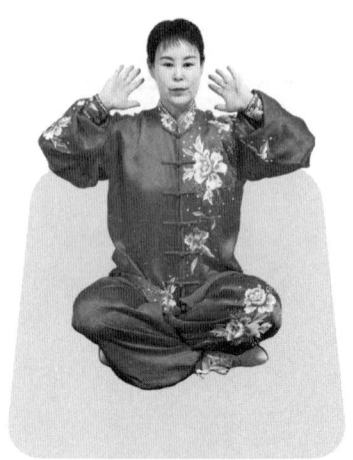

图 19/Figure 19

动作九：上动不停，两掌前伸按于腹前，掌心向下；目视前方。（图20）

Movement 9: Without a pause, bring both palms forward and press them down to the front of the abdomen, facing down. Eyes look ahead. (Figure 20)

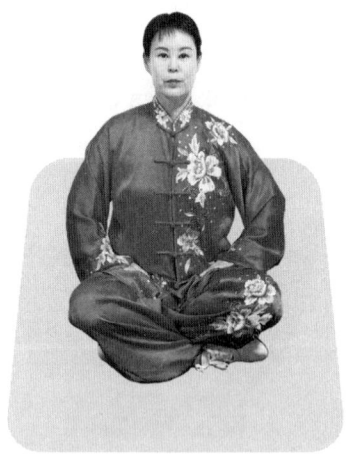

图 20/Figure 20

二、学练要领
II. Key Points

1. 呼吸时，要鼻吸鼻呼。

Breathe in and out through the nose.

2. 叩齿时，要掩实耳孔，静听默数，叩齿宜轻，略带咬劲，嘴唇轻闭。

When clicking the teeth, cover the ear holes tightly, listen and count silently. Click the teeth gently with a slight bite, lips lightly closed.

3. 鸣鼓时，食指要有弹力。

When sounding the drums, the index fingers should be elastic.

三、功理功用
III. Functions and Effects

1. 叩齿可坚固牙齿，防治牙科疾病。

Clicking the teeth can strengthen them and prevent dental diseases.

2. 叩齿可以对大脑进行轻度的刺激，对提高听力、预防耳鸣有积极作用。

Clicking the teeth can provide mild stimulation to the brain and has a positive effect on improving hearing and preventing tinnitus.

3. 鸣鼓可醒脑集神，耳聪目明。

Sounding the drums can refresh the mind and improve hearing and vision.

四、适宜症状
IV. Indications

1. 对龋齿等牙病有一定的防治作用。

It can prevent and treat dental diseases such as dental caries.

2. 可以预防和缓解伤风感冒、中风不语、肝气怒发、突然耳聋等症状。

It can prevent and alleviate symptoms such as cold, stroke, aphasia, liver *Qi* stagnation, and sudden deafness.

3. 对头昏、头痛、眼痛、肩背痛、颈椎病有较好的康复作用。

It is an aid to recovery from symptoms such as dizziness, headache, eye pain, shoulder and back pain, and cervical spondylosis.

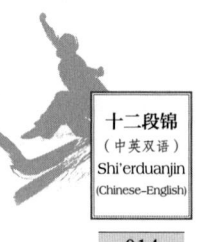

第三式　微撼天柱

Posture 3　Slightly Shake Heavenly Column

一、功法操作
I. Instructions

动作一：接上式，上体左转约 45 度，同时，两臂内旋成侧平举，掌心向后；目视左掌。（图 21）

Movement 1: Continuing from the end of the previous posture, turn your upper body approximately 45 degrees to the left. At the same time, rotate both arms inward and raise them to the sides of your body at shoulder level, palms facing back. Eyes look at the left palm. (Figure 21)

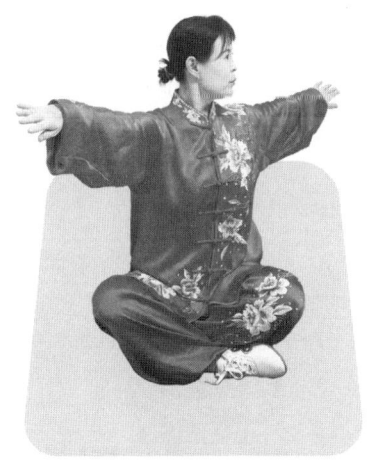

图 21/Figure 21

动作二：上动不停，上体向右转正，同时，两臂外旋平摆至体前约 45 度，掌心向下；目视前方。（图 22）

Movement 2: Without a pause, turn your upper body to face

forward. At the same time, rotate both arms outward and bring them inward to about 45 degrees in front of your body, palms facing down. Eyes look ahead. (Figure 22)

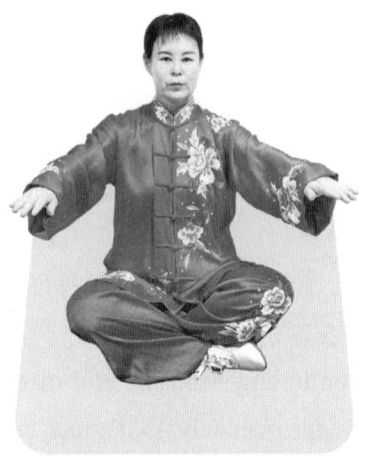

图 22/Figure 22

动作三：上动不停，两掌抱于体前，左掌在上，掌心向下，右掌在下，掌心向上，两掌心相对；目视前方。（图 23）

Movement 3: Without a pause, bring both palms together in front of your body as if holding a ball, with the left palm above and the right one below, facing each other. Eyes look ahead. (Figure 23)

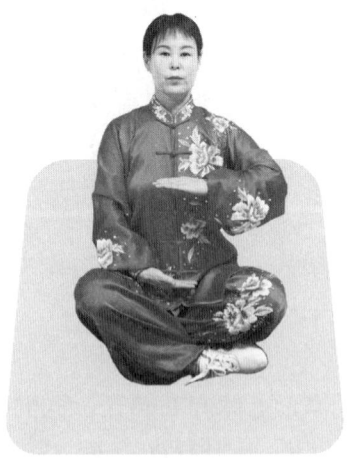

图 23/Figure 23

动作四：上动不停，左掌下按，两掌合于腹前；目视前方。（图24）

Movement 4: Without a pause, press the left palm down to join the right one in front of the abdomen. Eyes look ahead. (Figure 24)

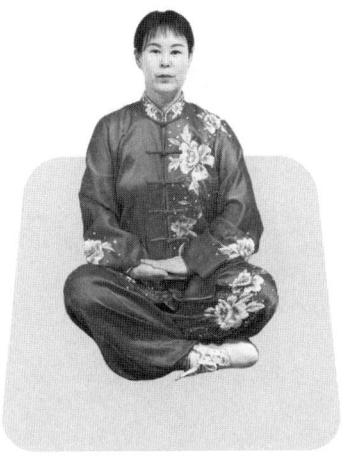

图 24/Figure 24

动作五：头向左转约90度，同时，两掌向右移至右大腿内侧；目视左侧。（图25）

Movement 5: Turn your head approximately 90 degrees to the left. At the same time, move both palms to the inner right thigh. Eyes look to the left. (Figure 25)

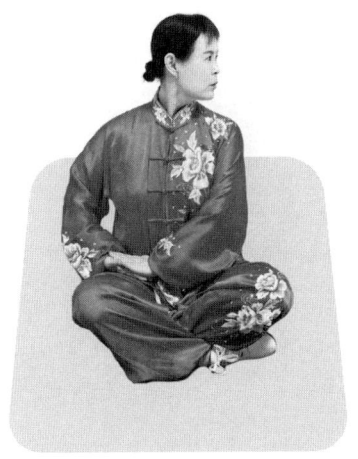

图 25/Figure 25

动作六：左肩下沉，左掌根向下压右掌；同时，向上抬下颏，稍停；目视左上方。（图26）

Movement 6: Lower the left shoulder and press the left palm down on the right palm. At the same time, raise the chin slightly. Pause for a while. Eyes look up to the left. (Figure 26)

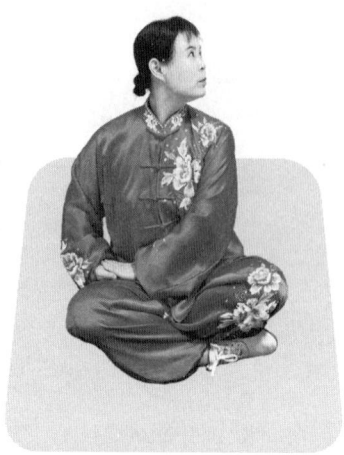

图26/Figure 26

动作七：身体姿势保持不变，下颏内收；目视左侧。（图27）

Movement 7: With the position of your body unchanged, tuck in the chin. Eyes look to the left. (Figure 27)

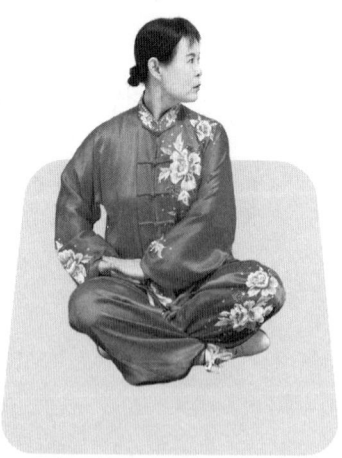

图27/Figure 27

动作八：头向右转约 90 度，面向体前，同时，两掌移至腹前；目视前方。（图 28）

Movement 8: Turn your head approximately 90 degrees to the right, facing forward. At the same time, move both palms to the front of the abdomen. Eyes look ahead. (Figure 28)

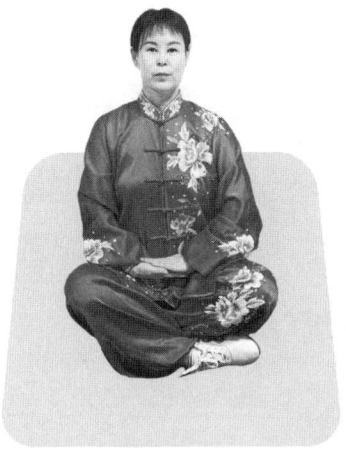

图 28/Figure 28

动作九：同动作一，唯左右相反。（图 29）

Movement 9: Repeat Movement 1, but with left and right reversed. (Figure 29)

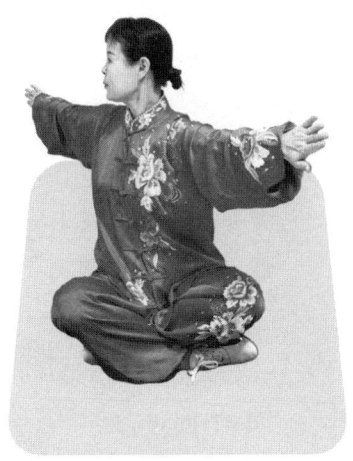

图 29/Figure 29

动作十：同动作二，唯左右相反。（图 30）

Movement 10: Repeat Movement 2, but with left and right reversed. (Figure 30)

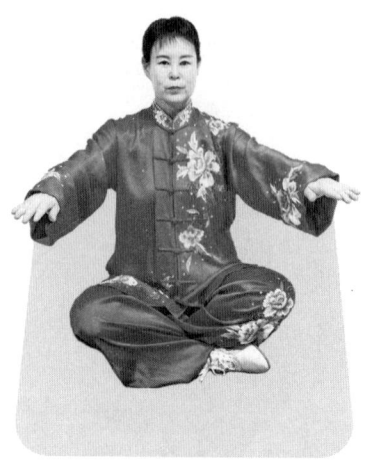

图 30/Figure 30

动作十一：同动作三，唯左右相反。（图 31）

Movement 11: Repeat Movement 3, but with left and right reversed. (Figure 31)

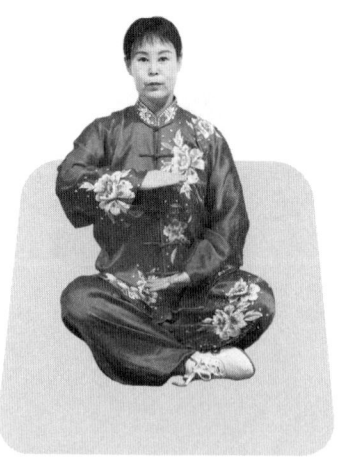

图 31/Figure 31

动作十二：同动作四，唯左右相反。（图 32）

Movement 12: Repeat Movement 4, but with left and right reversed. (Figure 32)

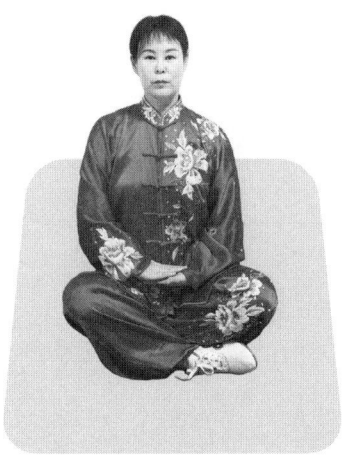

图 32/Figure 32

动作十三：同动作五，唯左右相反。（图 33）

Movement 13: Repeat Movement 5, but with left and right reversed. (Figure 33)

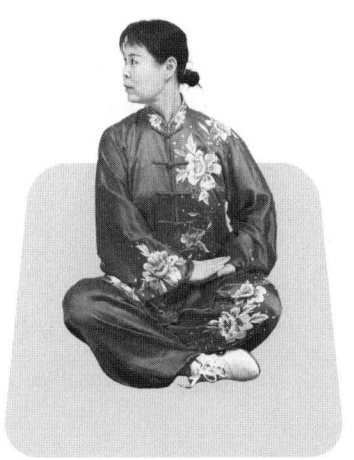

图 33/Figure 33

动作十四：同动作六，唯左右相反。（图 34）

Movement 14: Repeat Movement 6, but with left and right reversed. (Figure 34)

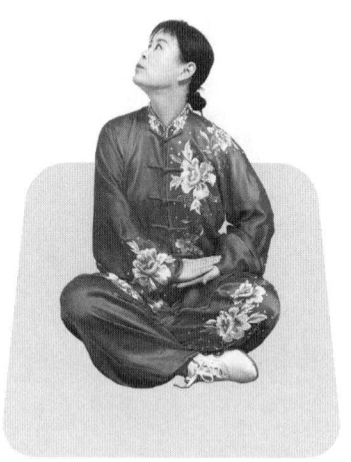

图 34/Figure 34

动作十五：同动作七，唯左右相反。（图 35）

Movement 15: Repeat Movement 7, but with left and right reversed. (Figure 35)

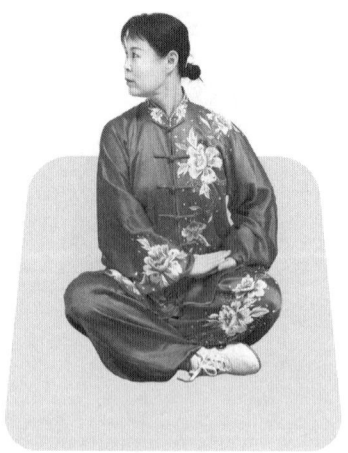

图 35/Figure 35

动作十六：同动作八，唯左右相反。（图 36）

Movement 16: Repeat Movement 8, but with left and right reversed. (Figure 36)

本式一左一右为 1 遍，共做 3 遍，接动作十七。

The movements on the left and the movements on the right form a round. Do three rounds, followed by Movement 17.

动作十七：两掌屈肘收于腰侧，掌心向内，指尖斜向下；目视前方。（图 37）

Movement 17: With the elbows bent, bring both palms to the sides of the waist, facing inward, fingers pointing diagonally downward. Eyes look ahead. (Figure 37)

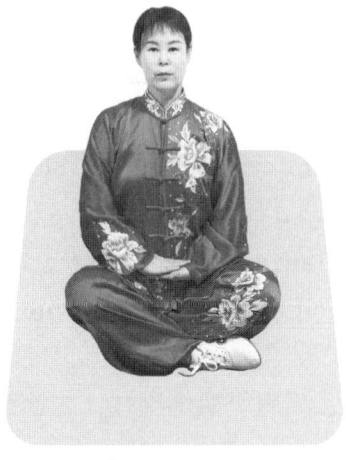
图 36/Figure 36

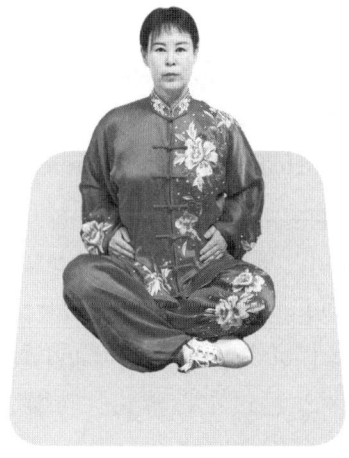
图 37/Figure 37

二、学练要领
II. Key Points

1. 转腰旋臂时，以腰带臂，沉肩坠肘、立身中正。

When turning the waist and rotating your arms, use the waist to lead the arms, shoulders and elbows sinking, your upper body straight.

2. 转头时，上体不动，立项竖脊；抬下颏时，稍用力，充分挤压大椎穴，颈项不可松懈断劲。

When turning your head, keep your upper body still, neck and spine erect. When raising the chin, use a little force to fully press *Dazhui* acupoint. The neck should not relax or lose power.

3. 抬头、收下颏、转头动作要清晰有序进行，不可同时完成。

Raising your head, tucking in the chin, and turning your head should be executed clearly and sequentially rather than simultaneously.

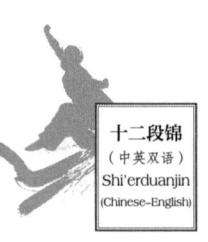

三、功理功用
III. Functions and Effects

1. "天柱"指整个颈椎。撼动天柱可刺激大椎穴，改善脑部的供血，增加血流量；调节手足三阳经和督脉，有散寒、除湿等功效。

"Heavenly column" refers to the entire cervical vertebra. Shaking the heavenly column can stimulate *Dazhui* acupoint, improve blood supply to the brain, increase blood flow, regulate the three *Yang* meridians of the hands and feet as well as *Du* Meridian, with the effects of dispelling cold and dampness.

2. 通过左右转头、转腰、旋臂、沉肩可锻炼脊柱，防治颈、肩、腰部位疾病。

By turning your head, waist, rotating the arms, and sinking the shoulders, the spine can be exercised to prevent diseases of the neck, shoulder, and waist.

四、适宜症状
IV. Indications

1. 可预防和改善风寒感冒引起的发热、打喷嚏、流涕、咳嗽等症状。

It can prevent and alleviate symptoms such as fever, sneezing, running nose, and cough caused by cold and flu.

2. 对颈椎病引起的颈椎不适、头疼、颈椎疼痛、活动受限、肢体麻木等症状有很好的改善作用。

It can alleviate the cervical discomfort, headache, cervical pain, limited mobility, and limb numbness caused by cervical spondylosis.

第四式 掌抱昆仑

Posture 4 Hold *Kunlun* in Hands

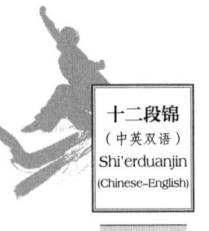

一、功法操作

I. Instructions

动作一：接上式，两肩后展，随之两掌前伸，直臂上举，掌心相对；目视前方。（图38）

Movement 1: Continuing from the end of the previous posture, spread the shoulders backward. Extend both palms forward and raise the arms straight up, palms facing each other. Eyes look ahead. (Figure 38)

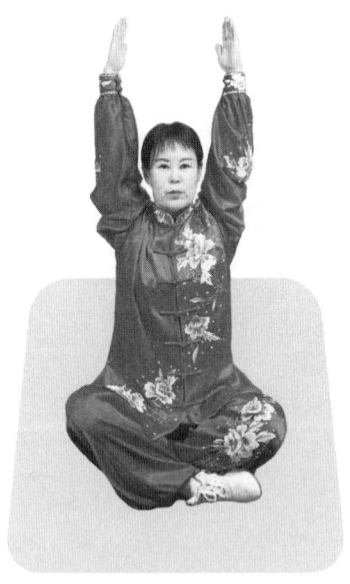

图 38/Figure 38

动作二：上动不停，两臂屈肘，十指交叉抱于脑后；目视前方。（图 39）

Movement 2: Without a pause, bend the elbows and cross the ten fingers to hold the back of your head. Eyes look ahead. (Figure 39)

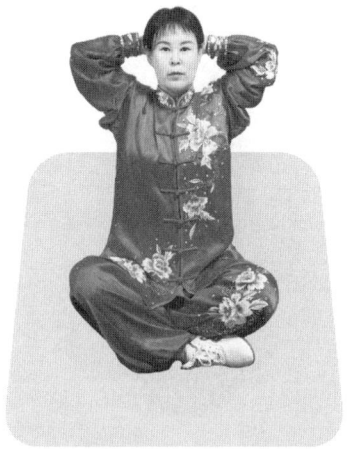

图 39/Figure 39

动作三：两掌抱头不动，上体左转约 45 度；目视左前方。（图 40）

Movement 3: Holding your head with both palms, turn your upper body about 45 degrees to the left. Eyes look to the left front. (Figure 40)

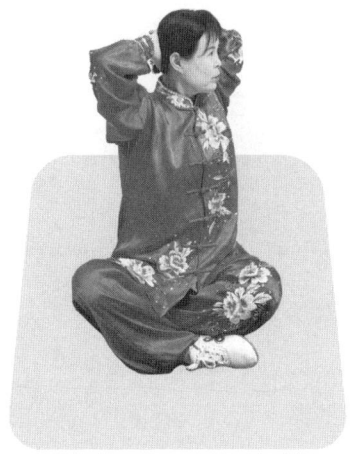

图 40/Figure 40

动作四：两掌抱头不动，上体右倾，抻拉左胁肋部；目视左斜上方。（图41）

Movement 4: Holding your head with both palms, tilt your upper body to the right, stretching the left ribcage. Eyes look to the upper left. (Figure 41)

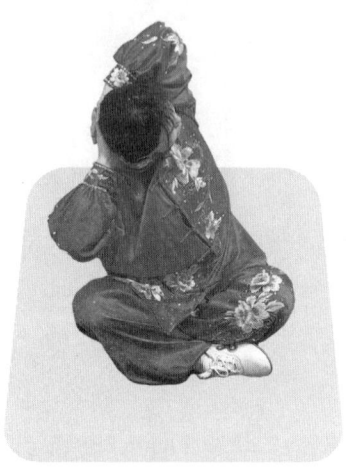

图 41/Figure 41

动作五：两掌抱头不动，上体直立；目视左前方。（图42）

Movement 5: Holding your head with both palms, straighten your upper body. Eyes look to the left front. (Figure 42)

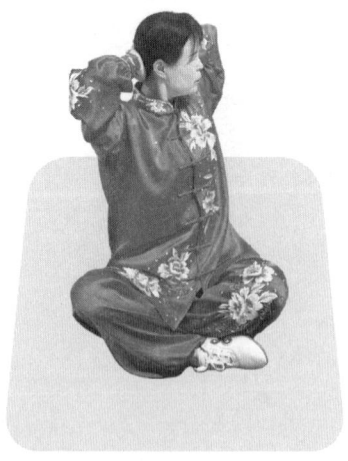

图 42/Figure 42

动作六：两掌抱头不动，上体向右转正；目视前方。（图43）

Movement 6: Holding your head with both palms, turn your upper body to face forward. Eyes look ahead. (Figure 43)

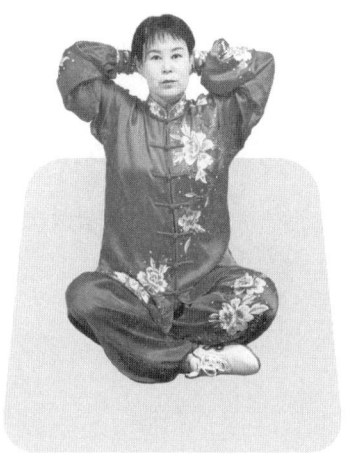

图43/Figure 43

动作七：同动作三，唯左右相反。（图44）

Movement 7: Repeat Movement 3, but with left and right reversed. (Figure 44)

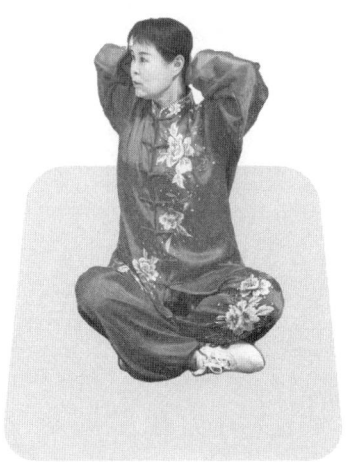

图44/Figure 44

动作八：同动作四，唯左右相反。（图45）

Movement 8: Repeat Movement 4, but with left and right reversed. (Figure 45)

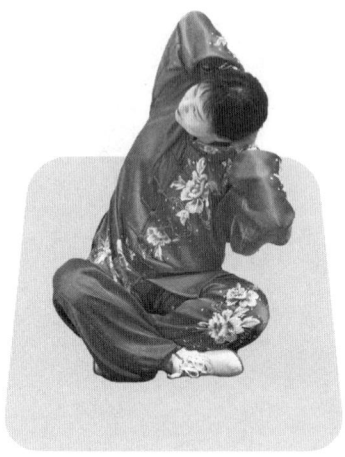

图45/Figure 45

动作九：同动作五，唯左右相反。（图46）

Movement 9: Repeat Movement 5, but with left and right reversed. (Figure 46)

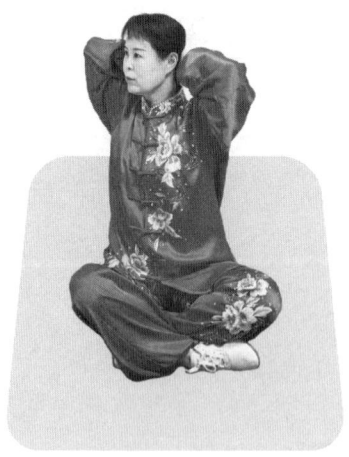

图46/Figure 46

动作十：同动作六，唯左右相反。（图 47）

Movement 10: Repeat Movement 6, but with left and right reversed. (Figure 47)

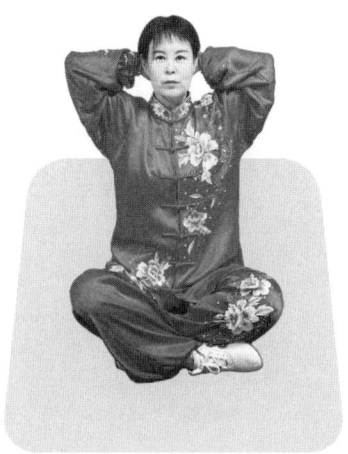

图 47/Figure 47

动作十一：两掌抱头不动，头向上抬起，与颈部有相对抗的争力；目视前上方。（图 48）

Movement 11: Holding your head with both palms, raise your head up with a contending force against the neck. Eyes look to the upper front. (Figure 48)

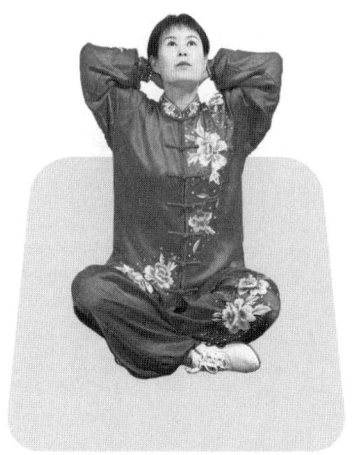

图 48/Figure 48

动作十二：向前合肘，随之下颏内收，两掌抱头稍向下推按；目视腹部。（图49）

Movement 12: Bring both elbows together forward, chin tucked in. Push your head slightly down with both palms. Eyes look at the abdomen. (Figure 49)

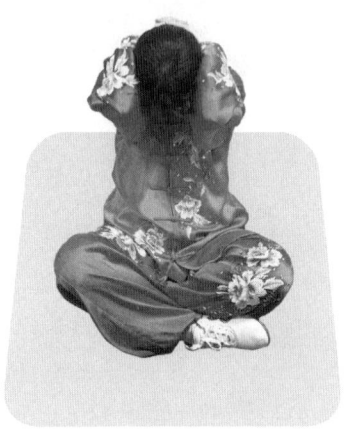

图 49/Figure 49

动作十三：两掌分开贴两颊下移，掌根贴下颏；目视前下方。（图50）

Movement 13: Separate the palms and move them down along the cheeks, with the bases of the palms pressed against the chin. Eyes look down to the front. (Figure 50)

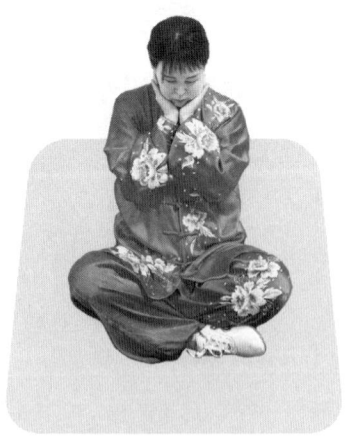

图 50/Figure 50

动作十四：上动不停，抬头，同时两掌上托下颏；目视上方。（图 51）

Movement 14: Without a pause, raise your head. At the same time, lift the chin with both palms. Eyes look up. (Figure 51)

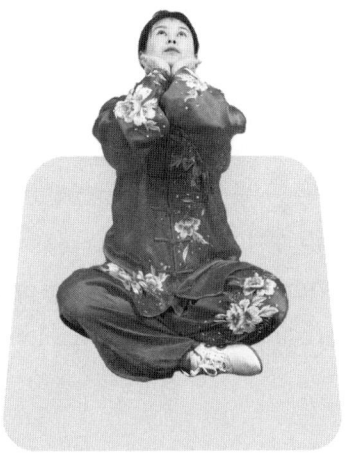

图 51/Figure 51

动作十五：下颏内收，颈部竖直，同时，两掌转掌心向下于肩前；目视前方。（图 52）

Movement 15: Tuck in the chin, neck erect. At the same time, turn both palms in front of the shoulders, facing down. Eyes look ahead. (Figure 52)

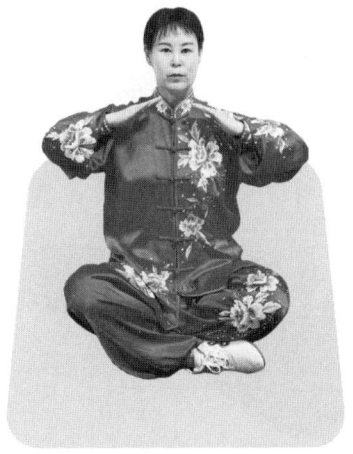

图 52/Figure 52

动作十六：两掌下按至腹前，臂外旋变指尖向前收于腰间；目视前方。（图53）

Movement 16: Press both palms down to the front of the abdomen, rotate both arms outward and bring the palms to the sides of the waist, fingers pointing forward. Eyes look ahead. (Figure 53)

以上动作共做3遍。第3遍结束时，接做动作十七。

Repeat the above movements three times, followed by Movement 17.

动作十七：身体姿势保持不变，两掌变握拳抱于腰间；目视前方。（图54）（图55拳）

Movement 17: With the position of your upper body unchanged, turn both palms into fists at the waist. Eyes look ahead. (Figure 54) (Figure 55 fist)

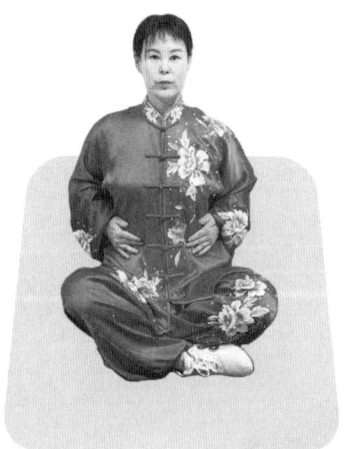
图53/Figure 53

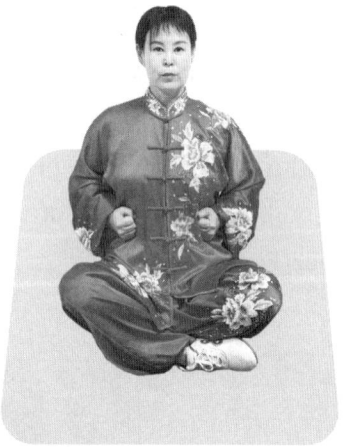
图54/Figure 54

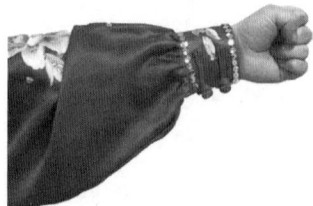
图55拳/Figure 55 fist

二、学练要领
II. Key Points

1. 抱头转体时，要充分向后展开肩和肘；左右侧倾身体时，异侧肘要充分上抬，充分抻拉两胁肋部。

When turning your body with the head held in hands, fully extend the shoulders and elbows backward. When tilting your upper body to the left or right, fully raise the opposite elbow, stretching the ribs on both sides.

2. 低头时，身体要中正、下颏要收紧；抬头时，要挺胸塌腰。

When lowering your head, keep your upper body upright and tuck in the chin tightly. When raising your head, lift the chest and sink the waist.

三、功理功用
III. Functions and Effects

1. 两手上举，可使三焦通畅、调和脾胃。

Raising both hands up can promote the function of triple energizer and regulate the spleen and stomach.

2. 身体左右侧倾可刺激肝经、胆经，起到疏肝利胆的作用。

Tilting your upper body to the left or right can stimulate the liver and gallbladder meridians, and have the effect of soothing the liver and promoting bile flow.

3. 两手抱头下拉可刺激督脉、膀胱经和背腧穴，调理相应脏腑。

Pushing your head down with both hands can stimulate *Du* and bladder meridians and *Beishu* acupoint, regulating the corresponding viscera.

4. 两手托下颏抬起，可刺激大椎穴，有解表散寒、通络止痛的作用。

Lifting the chin with both hands can stimulate *Dazhui* acupoint, with the effect of dispelling cold and alleviating pain by unblocking collaterals.

四、适宜症状
IV. Indications

有利于口干舌燥、咽喉肿痛、头疼、颈椎不适、胸闷不舒、两胁胀满、尿频、便秘等症状的预防和调治。

It can help to prevent and treat the symptoms such as dry mouth, sore throat, headache, cervical discomfort, chest tightness, distension of both sides of the ribcage, frequent urination, and constipation.

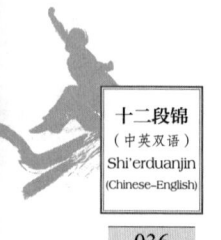

第五式　摇转辘轳

Posture 5　Rotate Arms like Windlass

一、功法操作
I. Instructions

动作一：接上式，两拳后移置于腰后肾俞穴处，拳心向后；目视前方。（图 56 正面、图 56 背面）

Movement 1: Continuing from the end of the previous posture, move both fists to *Shenshu* acupoints at the back of the waist, the hearts of fists facing backward. Eyes look ahead. (Figure 56 front, Figure 56 back)

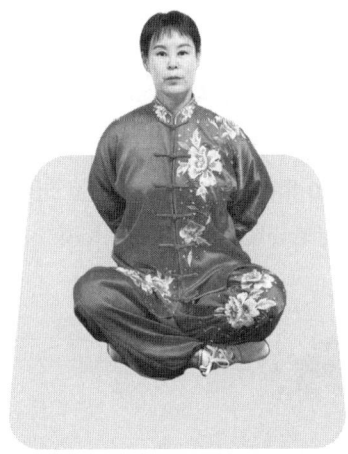   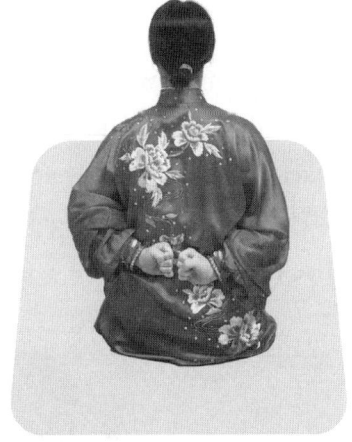

图 56 正面 /Figure 56 front　　图 56 背面 /Figure 56 back

动作二：上体左转约 45 度，同时，左拳屈腕上提，自腰后至左肩前，拳心向下，右拳位置保持不变；目视左拳。（图 57）

Movement 2: Turn your upper body approximately 45 degrees to the left. At the same time, raise the left fist with a flexed wrist from behind the waist to the front of the left shoulder, the heart of fist facing downward. The position of the right fist stays unchanged. Eyes look at the left fist. (Figure 57)

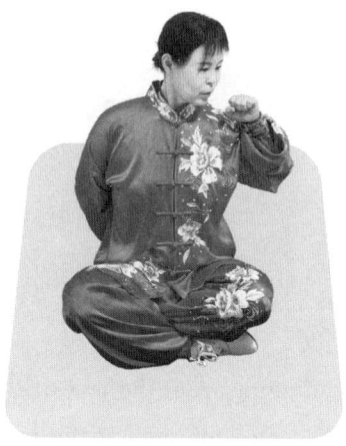

图 57/Figure 57

动作三：上动不停，上体右转，随之向左侧倾；同时，左腕上翘向左前方约 45 度前伸，肘关节微屈，右拳位置保持不变；目视左拳。（图 58）

Movement 3: Without a pause, turn your upper body to the right and then tilt it to the left. At the same time, with the left wrist flexed up, extend it approximately 45 degrees to the left front, elbow slightly bent. The position of the right fist stays unchanged. Eyes look at the left fist. (Figure 58)

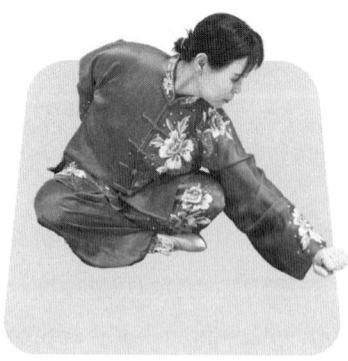

图 58/Figure 58

动作四：上动不停，上体左转至立身中正，同时，左拳回拉收至腰左侧，屈腕拳心向后，右拳位置保持不变；目视左拳。（图59）

Movement 4: Without a pause, turn your upper body to the left to an upright position. At the same time, bring the left fist back to the left side of the waist, wrist flexed, the heart of fist facing backward. The position of the right fist stays unchanged. Eyes look at the left fist. (Figure 59)

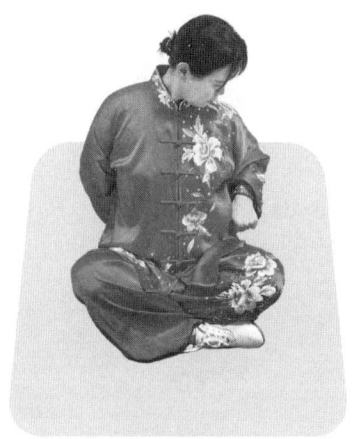

图 59/Figure 59

动作二至动作四，连续做6遍，为左摇转辘轳。第6遍结束时，接做动作五。

Repeat Movements 2 through 4 six times continuously, called "Rotate Left Arm like Windlass". After the sixth repetition, do Movement 5.

动作五：上体向右转正，左拳收至腰后肾俞穴处，拳心向后，右拳位置保持不变；目视前方。（图60）

Movement 5: Turn your upper body to the right, facing forward. Bring the left fist back to *Shenshu* acupoint at the back of the waist, the heart of fist facing backward. The position of the right fist stays unchanged. Eyes look ahead. (Figure 60)

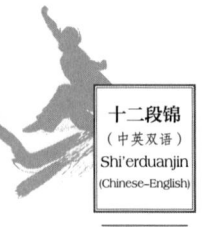

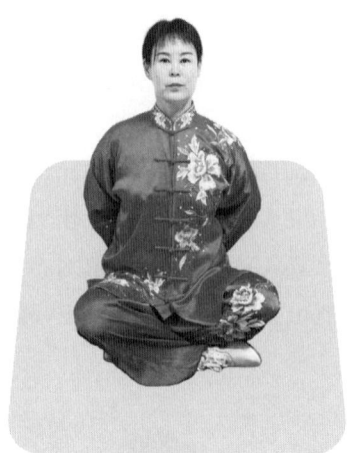

图 60/Figure 60

动作六：同动作二，唯左右相反。（图 61）

Movement 6: Repeat Movement 2, but with left and right reversed. (Figure 61)

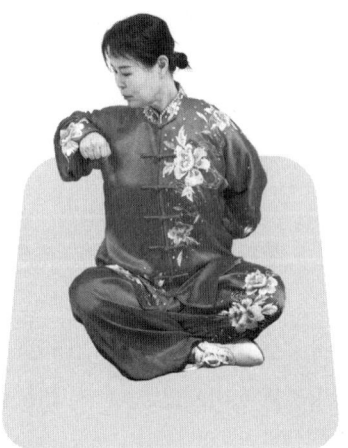

图 61/Figure 61

动作七：同动作三，唯左右相反。（图 62）

Movement 7: Repeat Movement 3, but with left and right reversed. (Figure 62)

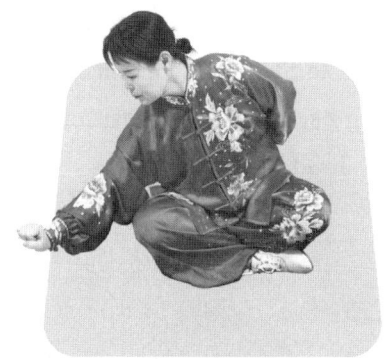

图 62/Figure 62

动作八：同动作四，唯左右相反。（图 63）

Movement 8: Repeat Movement 4, but with left and right reversed. (Figure 63)

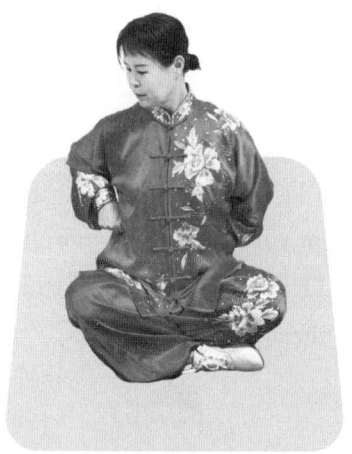

图 63/Figure 63

动作六至动作八，连续做 6 遍，为右摇转辘轳。第 6 遍结束时，接做动作九。

Repeat Movements 6 through 8 six times continuously, called "Rotate Right Arm like Windlass". After the sixth repetition, do Movement 9.

动作九：上体向左转正，右拳收至腰后肾俞穴处，拳心向后，左拳位置保持不变；目视前方。（图 64）

Movement 9: Turn your upper body to the left, facing forward. Bring the right fist back to *Shenshu* acupoint at the back of the waist, the heart of fist facing backward. The position of the left fist stays unchanged. Eyes look ahead. (Figure 64)

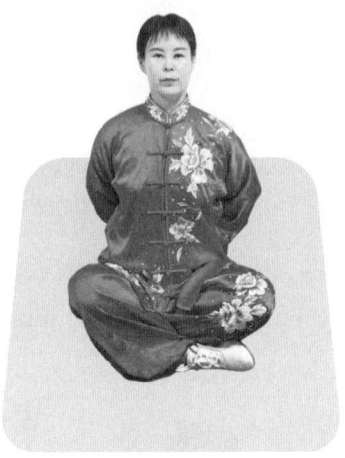

图 64/Figure 64

动作十：身体中正，立项竖脊，展肩扩胸，两拳位置保持不变；目视前方。（图 65）

Movement 10: With your upper body upright, erect the neck and spine, expand the shoulders and chest. The positions of the fists stays unchanged. Eyes look ahead. (Figure 65)

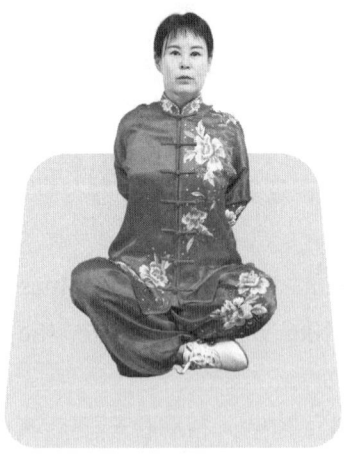

图 65/Figure 65

动作十一：上动不停，保持身体中正，两肩同时向上提，两拳位置保持不变；目视前方。（图 66）

Movement 11: Without a pause, keep your upper body upright. Raise both shoulders simultaneously, the positions of the fists unchanged. Eyes look ahead. (Figure 66)

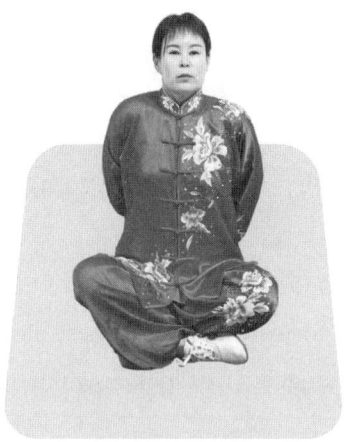

图 66/Figure 66

动作十二：上动不停，两肩再向前合肩含胸，两拳位置保持不变；目视前下方。（图 67）

Movement 12: Without a pause, bring both shoulders forward together, chest drawn in. The positions of the fists stays unchanged. Eyes look down to the front. (Figure 67)

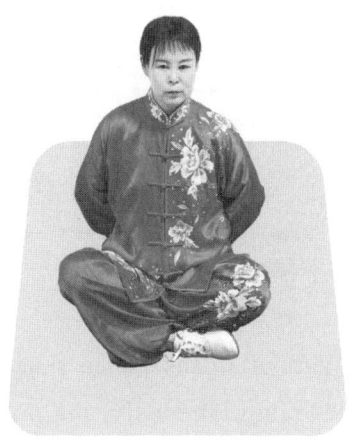

图 67/Figure 67

动作十至动作十二，双肩向前绕环连续做6遍。第6遍结束时，接做动作十三。

Do Movements 10 through 12 six times continuously, circling the shoulders forward each time. After the sixth repetition, do Movement 13.

动作十三：两肩放松下沉，两拳位置保持不变，立项竖脊，正身端坐；目视前方。（图68）

Movement 13: Relax and sink both shoulders, with the positions of the fists unchanged. Erect the neck and spine, sitting upright. Eyes look ahead. (Figure 68)

动作十四：接上动，两肩向前合肩含胸，两拳位置保持不变；目视前下方。（图69）

Movement 14: Continuing from the end of the previous movement, bring both shoulders forward together, chest drawn in. The positions of the fists stays unchanged. Eyes look down to the front. (Figure 69)

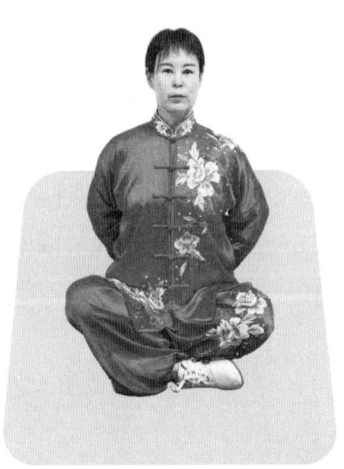 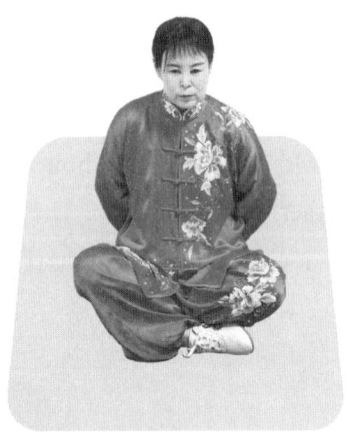

图68/Figure 68　　　　　图69/Figure 69

动作十五：上动不停，保持身体中正，两肩同时向上提，两拳位置保持不变；目视前方。（图70）

Movement 15: Without a pause, keep your upper body upright. Raise both shoulders simultaneously, the positions of the fists unchanged. Eyes look ahead. (Figure 70)

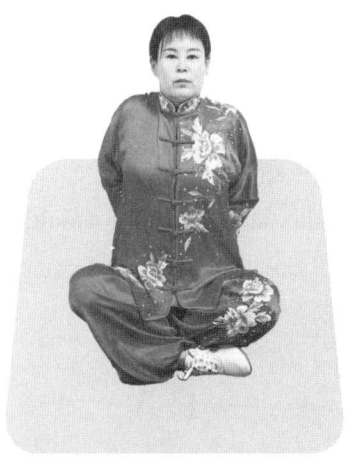

图 70/Figure 70

动作十六：上动不停，立项竖脊，展肩扩胸，两拳位置保持不变；目视前方。（图 71）

Movement 16: Without a pause, erect the neck and spine, expand the shoulders and chest. The positions of the fists stays unchanged. Eyes look ahead. (Figure 71)

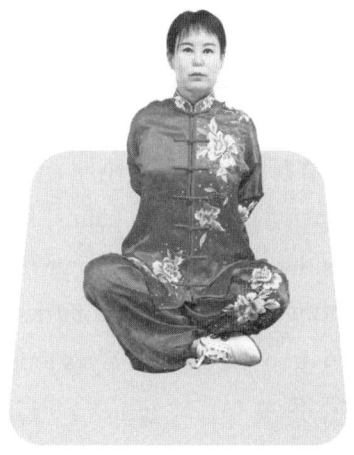

图 71/Figure 71

动作十四至动作十六，双肩向后绕环连续做 6 遍。第 6 遍结束时，接做动作十七。

Do Movements 14 through 16 six times continuously, circling the shoulders backward each time. After the sixth repetition, do Movement 17.

动作十七：两肩放松下沉，两拳位置保持不变，立项竖脊，正身端坐；目视前方。（图 72）

Movement 17: Relax and sink both shoulders, with the positions of the fists unchanged. Erect the neck and spine, sitting upright. Eyes look ahead. (Figure 72)

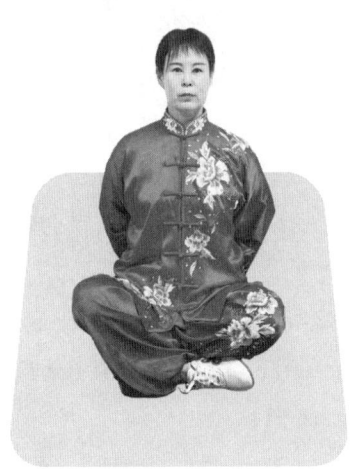

图 72/Figure 72

动作十八：两拳变掌，指尖向下，两虎口分别轻贴两肋上提至肩上，指尖向内，掌背向上，沉肩坠肘；目视前方。（图 73）

Movement 18: Open the fists into palms, fingers pointing down. Raise the palms above the shoulders, pressing *Hukou* against the ribs, with the fingers pointing inward and the backs of palms facing up. Sink the shoulders and drop the elbows. Eyes look ahead. (Figure 73)

动作十九：两手不动，上体左转约 90 度；目视前方。（图 74）

Movement 19: With the position of both hands in place, turn your upper body approximately 90 degrees to the left. Eyes look ahead. (Figure 74)

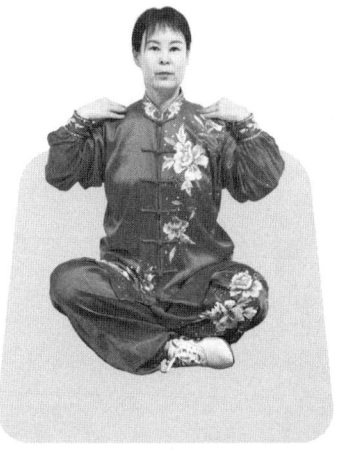 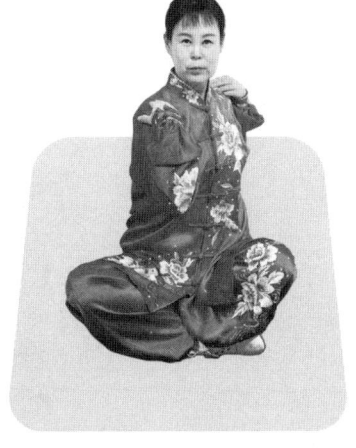

图 73/Figure 73　　　　　图 74/Figure 74

动作二十：上动不停，以肩为轴，右臂前摆，同时，左臂后摆；目视前方。（图 75）

Movement 20: Without a pause, rotate the right arm forward and the left arm backward around the shoulders as axes. Eyes look ahead. (Figure 75)

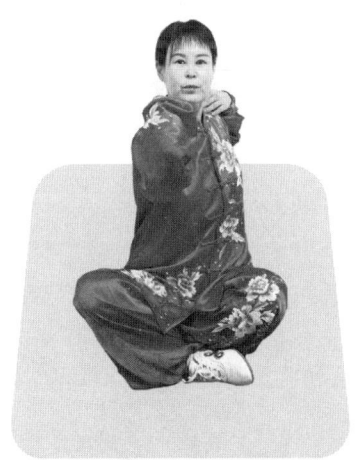

图 75/Figure 75

动作二十一：上动不停，上体向右转正，两臂继续上摆，肘尖向上；目视前方。（图 76）

Movement 21: Without a pause, turn your upper body to the right, facing forward. Continue to rotate both arms upward, elbows pointing up. Eyes look ahead. (Figure 76)

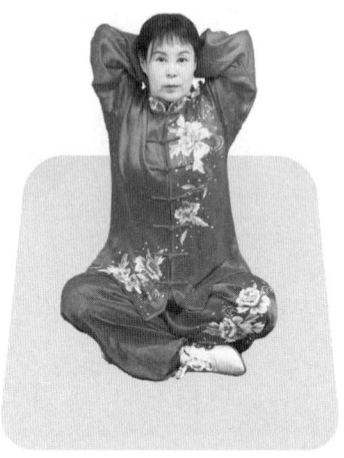

图 76/Figure 76

动作二十二：上动不停，上体向右转，左臂向前下摆，右臂向后下摆；目视前方。（图 77）

Movement 22: Without a pause, turn your upper body further to the right, rotating the left arm down to the front and the right arm down to the back. Eyes look ahead. (Figure 77)

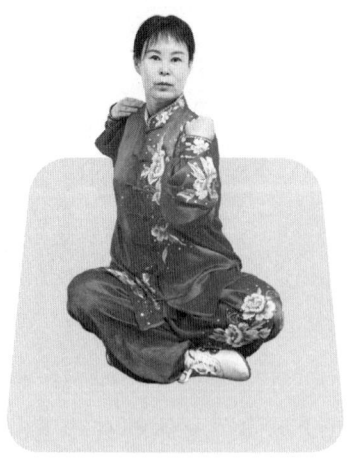

图 77/Figure 77

动作二十三：上动不停，上体向左转正，两臂下落，肘尖向下；目视前方。（图 78）

Movement 23: Without a pause, turn your upper body to the left, facing forward. Lower both arms, elbows pointing down. Eyes look ahead. (Figure 78)

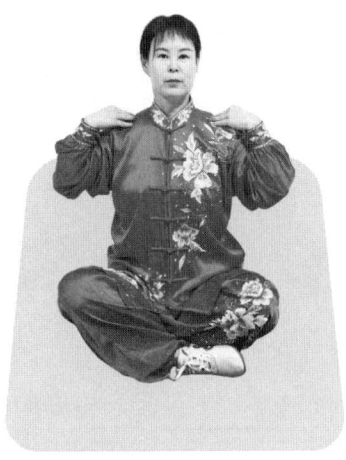

图 78/Figure 78

动作十九至动作二十三，前后交叉绕肩连续做 6 遍。第 6 遍结束时，接做动作二十四。

Do Movements 19 through 23 six times continuously, crisscross-rotating the arms forward and backward around the shoulders. After the sixth repetition, do Movement 24.

动作二十四：同动作十九，唯左右相反。（图 79）

Movement 24: Repeat Movement 19, but with left and right reversed. (Figure 79)

动作二十五：同动作二十，唯左右相反。（图 80）

Movement 25: Repeat Movement 20, but with left and right reversed. (Figure 80)

动作二十六：同动作二十一，唯左右相反。（图 81）

Movement 26: Repeat Movement 21, but with left and right reversed. (Figure 81)

动作二十七：同动作二十二，唯左右相反。（图 82）

Movement 27: Repeat Movement 22, but with left and right reversed. (Figure 82)

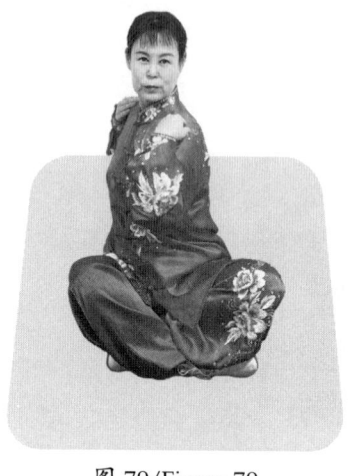
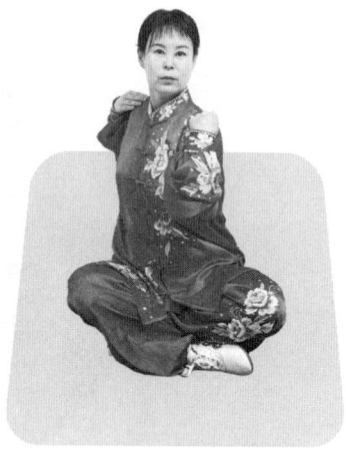

图 79/Figure 79　　　　图 80/Figure 80

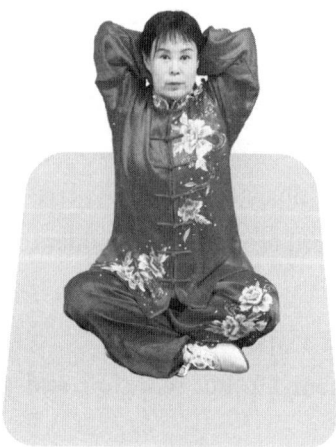
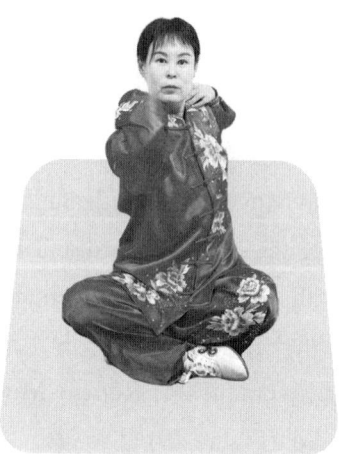

图 81/Figure 81　　　　图 82/Figure 82

动作二十八：同动作二十三，唯左右相反。（图 83）

Movement 28: Repeat Movement 23, but with left and right reversed. (Figure 83)

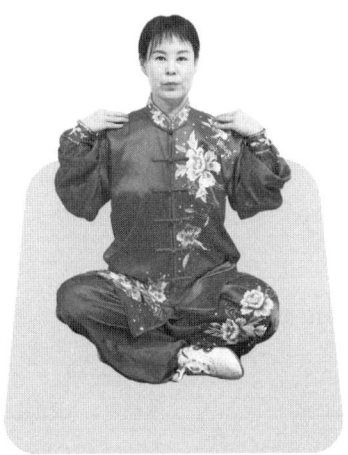

图 83/Figure 83

动作二十四至动作二十八，前后交叉绕肩连续做 6 遍。

Do Movements 24 through 28 six times continuously, crisscross-rotating the arms forward and backward around the shoulders.

二、学练要领
II. Key Points

1. 单臂摇转辘轳时，转腰、顺肩、臂前送、坐腕、臂回拉、屈肘、提腕要依次协调连贯完成动作。

When rotating one arm like windlass, turning the waist, forwarding the shoulder, extending the arm forward, flexing the wrist up, bringing the arm back, bending the elbow, and raising the wrist should be performed in sequence and in a coordinated and continuous manner.

2. 双肩前后绕环时，食指根节点揉肾腧穴，绕肩要圆活连贯。

When rotating the shoulders forward and backward, use the bases of index fingers to massage *Shenshu* acupoints. The rotation of the shoulders should be smooth and continuous.

3. 前后交叉绕肩时，以腰带臂绕立圆，两肘前后摆动要协调一致。

When crisscross-rotating the arms around the shoulders, use the waist to lead the arms in making vertical circles. The forward and backward motion of the arms should be coordinated.

三、功理功用
III. Functions and Effects

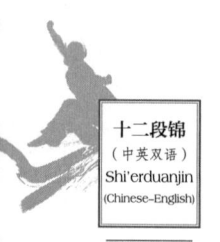

1. 本式动作可刺激手三阴三阳经、督脉、膀胱经、背俞穴，调理相应脏腑，有畅通心肺、益肾助阳的功效。

This posture can stimulate the three *Yin* and three *Yang* meridians of the hands, *Du* and bladder meridians, and *Beishu* acupoint. It can regulate the corresponding viscera, promoting cardiovascular and lung health, with the effect of tonifying the kidneys and supporting *Yang*.

2. 可强壮腰脊，防治肩部与颈椎疾患。

It can strengthen the waist and spine, and prevent shoulder and cervical spine disorders.

四、适宜症状
IV. Indications

1. 有利于缓解肩、肘、腕、颈、背、腰等部位的肌肉疼痛。

It can alleviate muscle pain in the shoulders, elbows, wrists, neck, back and waist.

2. 有利于心脏、脾脏、肺脏、肝脏，肾脏和膀胱等部位疾病的预防和缓解。

It can prevent and relieve diseases in the heart, spleen, lungs, liver, kidneys and bladder.

第六式 托天按顶

Posture 6 Hold Up Heaven and Press Crown

一、功法操作
I. Instructions

动作一：接上式，身体姿势保持不变，两肘上提与肩平；目视前方。（图 84）

Movement 1: Continuing from the end of the previous posture, with the position of your upper body unchanged, lift the elbows to shoulder level. Eyes look ahead. (Figure 84)

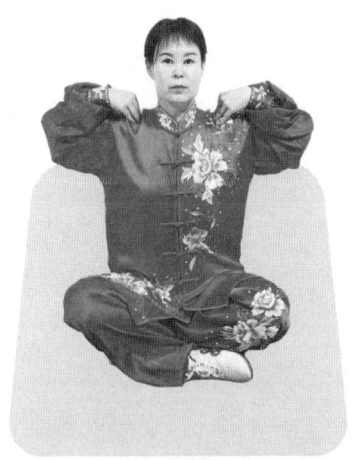

图 84/Figure 84

动作二：上动不停，身体姿势保持不变，两手虎口贴肋下插至身后髋关节处；目视前方。（图 85）

Movement 2: Without a pause, the position of your upper body stays unchanged. Move the palms down, *Hukou* against the ribs, to the buttocks. Eyes look ahead. (Figure 85)

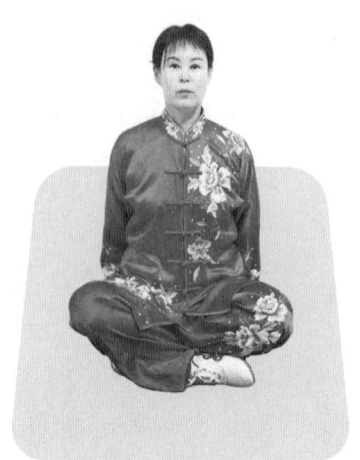

图 85/Figure 85

动作三：上动不停，身体姿势保持不变，两臂外旋，两掌心贴大腿外侧移至膝关节处，掌背向外；目视前下方。（图 86）

Movement 3: Without a pause, the position of your upper body stays unchanged. With both arms rotating outward, move the palms along the outer thighs to the knees, facing inward. Eyes look down to the front. (Figure 86)

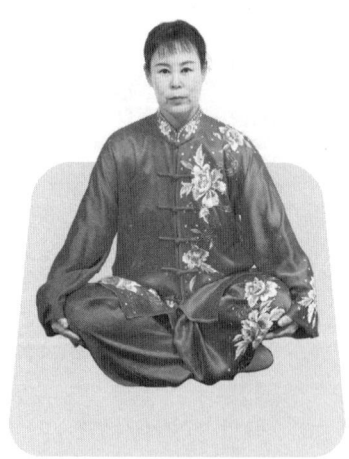

图 86/Figure 86

动作四：上动不停，身体姿势保持不变，两掌向上托膝，两膝移至两肋前，两脚位置不动；目视前下方。（图 87）

Movement 4: Without a pause, the position of your upper body stays unchanged. Lift the knees with both palms up to the ribs. Keep the feet in place. Eyes look down to the front. (Figure 87)

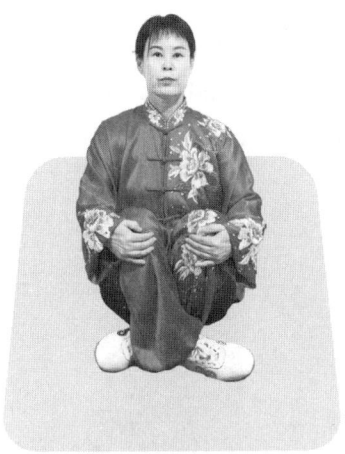

图 87/Figure 87

动作五：上动不停，右腿前伸，脚尖向上，膝关节微屈，左膝放松；目视右脚。（图 88）

Movement 5: Without a pause, extend the right leg forward, toes up, knee slightly bent. Relax the left knee. Eyes look at the right foot. (Figure 88)

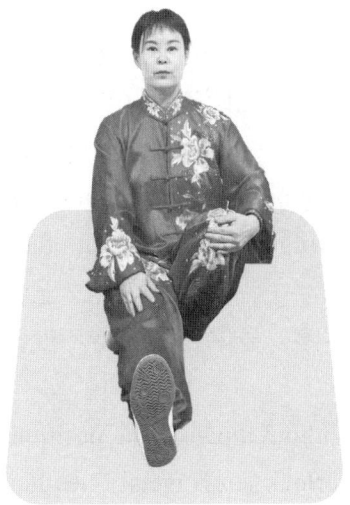

图 88/Figure 88

动作六：身体姿势保持不变，左脚前伸，两腿自然伸展，脚尖向上；同时两手轻扶膝关节，掌心向下，指尖斜向前；目视脚尖。（图89）

Movement 6: With the position of your upper body unchanged, extend the left foot forward. Stretch the legs naturally, toes up. At the same time, gently put your hands on the knees, palms facing down, fingers pointing diagonally forward. Eyes look at the toes. (Figure 89)

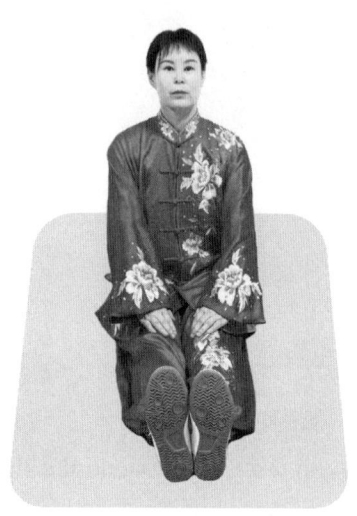

图89/Figure 89

动作七：上动不停，立身中正，两臂外旋，两掌收至腹前，指尖相对，掌心向上；目视前下方。（图90）

Movement 7: Without a pause, keep your upper body upright. With both arms rotating outward, bring both palms to the front of the abdomen, facing up, fingers pointing each other. Eyes look down to the front. (Figure 90)

动作八：上动不停，身体姿势保持不变，十指交叉；目视前下方。（图91）

Movement 8: Without a pause, the position of your upper body stays unchanged. Interlock ten fingers. Eyes look down to the front. (Figure 91)

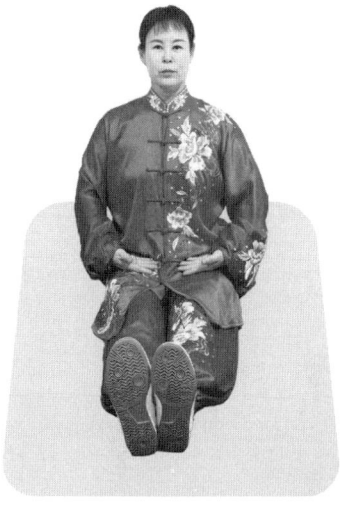
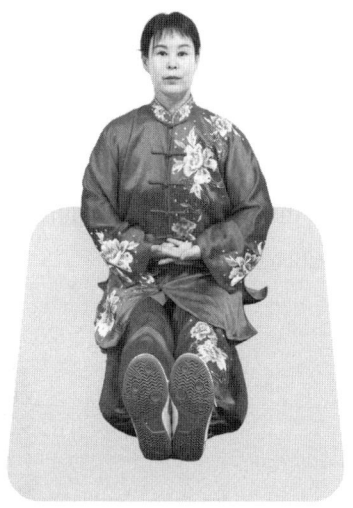

图 90/Figure 90　　　　　图 91/Figure 91

动作九：身体姿势保持不变，两手上托至胸部，掌心向上；目视前方。（图92）

Movement 9: With the position of your upper body unchanged, raise both hands to the chest, palms facing upward. Eyes look ahead. (Figure 92)

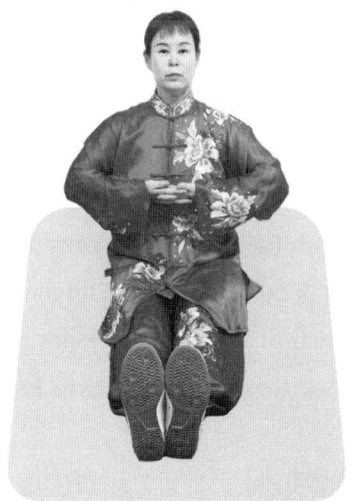

图 92/Figure 92

动作十：上动不停，身体保持立身中正，两臂内旋，翻掌直臂上托；同时，膝关节挺直，脚面绷平；目视前方。（图93）

Movement 10: Without a pause, keep your upper body upright. With both arms rotating inward, turn over the palms and raise them up. At the same time, straighten the knees and flatten the insteps. Eyes look ahead. (Figure 93)

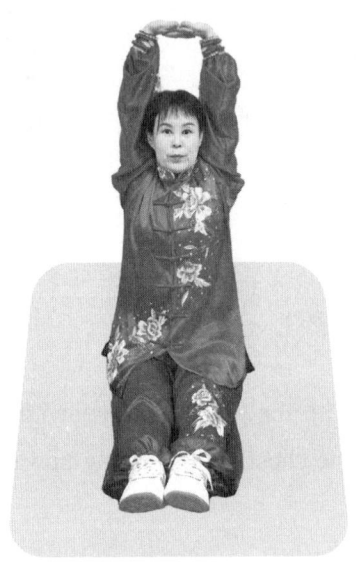

图93/Figure 93

动作十一：身体姿势保持不变，沉肩屈肘，两掌心翻转向下落至头顶，两手稍用力下压；同时两脚尖向上勾紧；目视前下方。（图94）

Movement 11: With the position of your upper body unchanged, sink the shoulders and bend the elbows. Flip the palms downward and lower them to the crown of the head, pressing it with slight force. At the same time, hook the toes up tightly. Eyes look down to the front. (Figure 94)

动作十二：身体姿势保持不变，两臂内旋，两掌心翻转向上，直臂上托；同时，膝关节挺直，脚面绷平；目视前方。（图95）

Movement 12: With the position of your upper body unchanged, rotate both arms inward, flip the palms up and raise them. At the same time, straighten the knees and flatten the insteps. Eyes look ahead. (Figure 95)

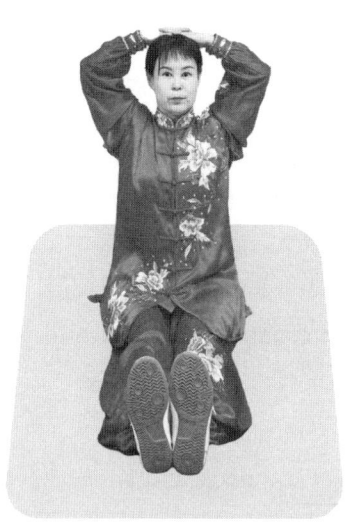

图 94/Figure 94

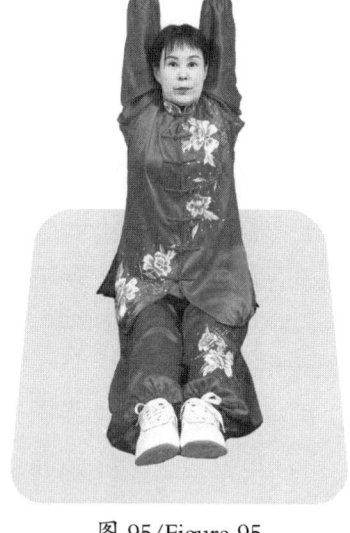

图 95/Figure 95

动作十三：身体姿势保持不变，沉肩屈肘，两掌心翻转向下落至头顶，两手稍用力下压；同时两脚尖向上勾紧；目视前下方。（图96）

Movement 13: With the position of your upper body unchanged, sink the shoulders and bend the elbows. Flip the palms downward and lower them to the crown of the head, pressing it with slight force. At the same time, hook the toes up tightly. Eyes look down to the front. (Figure 96)

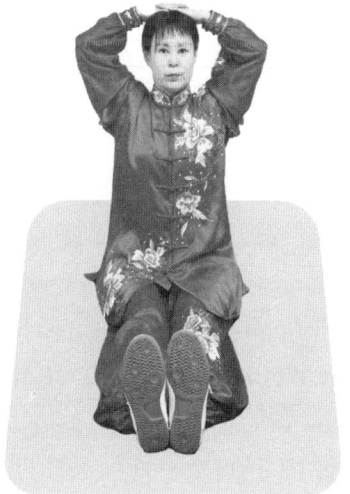

图 96/Figure 96

两掌上托下按为1遍，共做9遍。

Raising the palms up and pressing them down form a round. Do nine rounds.

二、学练要领
II. Key Points

1. 两掌上托时，躯干要保持直立，两臂要垂直地面，充分伸展腰臂，抻拉两胁肋部。

When raising both palms, keep your torso upright, arms perpendicular to the ground. Fully extend the waist and arms, stretching the rib cage.

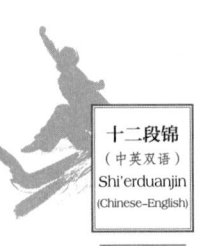

2. 两掌下按时，立项竖脊，身体中正。

When lowering both palms, erect the neck and spine, keeping your upper body upright.

3. 勾起和绷平脚面时，用力要充分，膝关节要伸展。

When hooking the toes up or flattening the insteps, apply sufficient force and extend the knees.

三、功理功用
III. Functions and Effects

1. 伸脚、勾脚可分别刺激足三阴三阳经，疏通经脉，促进气血运行。

Flattening the insteps and hooking the toes up can stimulate and dredge the three *Yin* and three *Yang* meridians of the feet, promoting the flow of *Qi* and blood.

2. 向上抻拉脊柱、两胁肋部和肩颈部，可调理三焦，疏肝利胆。

Stretching up the spine, ribcage, shoulders and neck can regulate the triple energizer and soothes the liver and gallbladder.

四、适宜症状
IV. Indications

1. 有利于肺部炽热、腹部胀满、两胁疼痛、大小便不利等症状的预防和调治。

It can help to prevent and treat symptoms such as lung heat, abdominal distension, pain in the ribcages, and urinary and fecal difficulties.

2. 有利于缓解颈、肩、肘、腕等部位的肌肉疼痛。

It can relieve muscle pain in the neck, shoulders, elbows and wrists.

第七式　俯身攀足

Posture 7　Bend to Touch Feet

一、功法操作
I. Instructions

动作一：接上式，身体姿势保持不变，两手分开直臂上举，掌心相对，踝关节放松，脚尖向上；目视前方。（图 97）

Movement 1: Continuing from the end of the previous posture, with the position of your upper body unchanged, separate the palms and lift them straight up, facing each other. Relax the ankles, toes up. Eyes look ahead. (Figure 97)

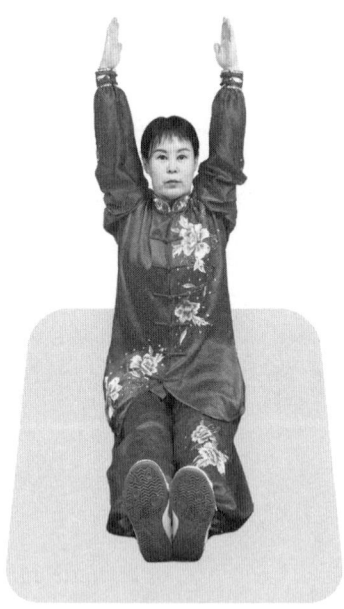

图 97/Figure 97

动作二：上动不停，上体前俯不超过 45 度，同时，两手前伸下落，抓握两脚掌，两肘自然伸展，拇指压于脚面；目视脚尖。（图 98）

Movement 2: Without a pause, bend your upper body forward by no more than 45 degrees. At the same time, stretch the hands forward and downward to grab the soles of the feet and press the thumbs onto the insteps, elbows naturally extending. Eyes look at the toes. (Figure 98)

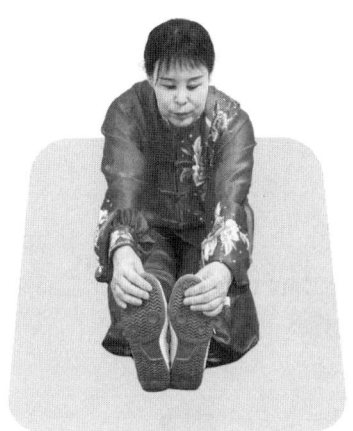

图 98/Figure 98

动作三：两手向身体方向回拉脚尖，脚尖勾紧，挺膝、塌腰、抬头，动作稍停；目视前上方。（图 99）

Movement 3: Pull the toes toward your body with both hands, hooking the toes up tightly. Straighten the knees, push the waist forward, and raise your head. Pause for a while. Eyes look up to the front. (Figure 99)

动作四：两手、两腿与腰脊姿势保持不变，下颌内收，抻拉脖颈，动作稍停；目视膝关节。（图 100）

Movement 4: With the positions of the hands, legs, and waist unchanged, tuck in the chin and stretch the neck. Pause for a while. Eyes look at the knees. (Figure 100)

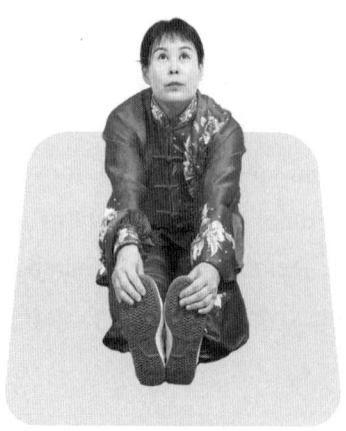
图 99/Figure 99

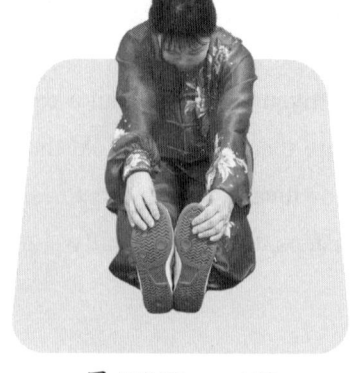
图 100/Figure 100

动作五：身体姿势保持不变，两手松开变掌扶于膝关节处，掌心向下；目视前方。（图101）

Movement 5: With the position of your upper body unchanged, open the hands into palms to rest on both knees, facing down. Eyes look ahead. (Figure 101)

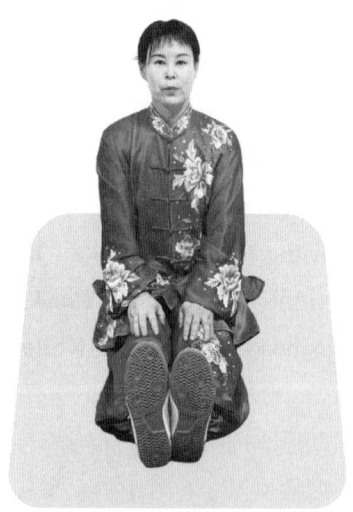
图 101/Figure 101

动作六：上体立起，颈部竖直，同时，两掌沿腿屈肘回收，经腰间向后向侧摆起，掌心向后；目视前方。（图102）

Movement 6: Straighten your upper body, neck erect. At the same time, draw both hands back along the legs to the waist, elbows bent, then swing the arms backward and to the sides, palms facing back. Eyes look ahead. (Figure 102)

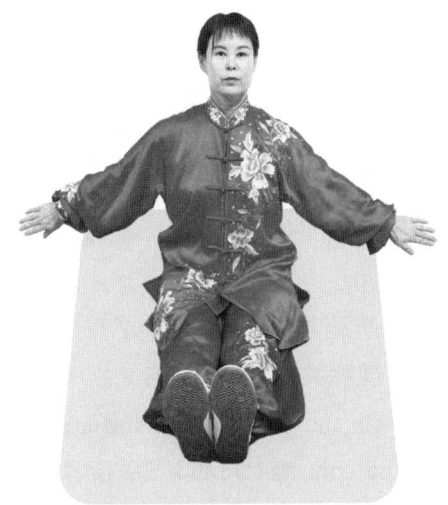

图 102/Figure 102

动作七：上动不停，上体前俯不超过 45 度，同时，两臂外旋，两掌弧形前摆，抓握脚掌，拇指压于脚面；目视脚尖。（图 103）

Movement 7: Without a pause, bend your upper body forward by no more than 45 degrees. At the same time, with both arms rotating outward, swing the palms forward in an arc to grasp the soles of the feet, thumbs pressing on the insteps. Eyes look at the toes. (Figure 103)

动作八：两手向身体方向回拉脚尖，脚尖勾紧，挺膝、塌腰、抬头，动作稍停；目视前上方。（图 104）

Movement 8: Pull the toes toward your body with both hands, hooking the toes up tightly. Straighten the knees, push the waist forward, and raise your head. Pause for a while. Eyes look up to the front. (Figure 104)

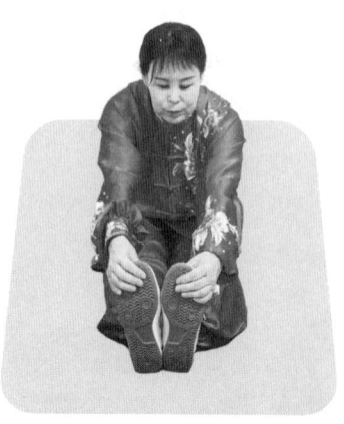 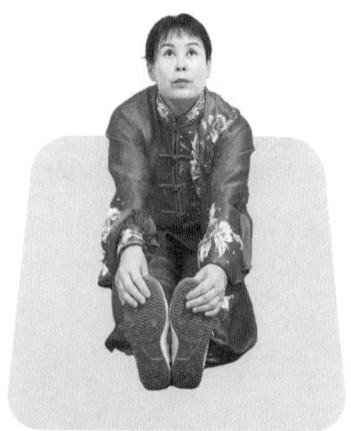

图 103/Figure 103　　　　图 104/Figure 104

动作九：两手、两腿与腰脊姿势保持不变，下颌内收，抻拉脖颈，动作稍停；目视膝关节。（图 105）

Movement 9: With the positions of the hands, legs, and waist unchanged, tuck in the chin and stretch the neck. Pause for a while. Eyes look at the knees. (Figure 105)

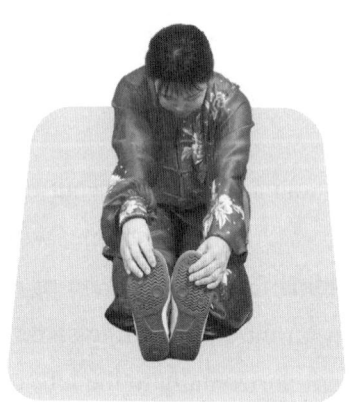

图 105/Figure 105

重复动作五至动作九 4 遍，抬头和收下颌动作共做 6 遍。第 6 遍结束时，接做动作十。

Repeat Movements 5 through 9 four times, with a total of six repetitions for raising your head and tucking in the chin. After the sixth repetition, do Movement 10.

动作十：上体立起，颈部竖直，同时两手松开扶于膝关节处；目视前方。（图106）

Movement 10: Straighten your upper body, neck erect. At the same time, loosen both hands to rest on the knees. Eyes look ahead. (Figure 106)

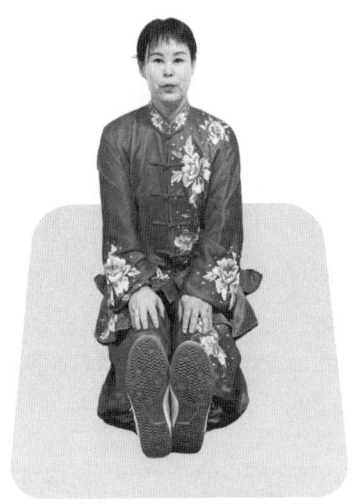

图106/Figure 106

动作十一：左臂外旋，掌心翻转向上，向右平行画弧，同时，右掌掌心向下，从左臂上方向左平行画弧，两臂合于腹前；目视前方。（图107）

Movement 11: Rotate the left arm outward, turning the palm up, and arc it horizontally to the right. At the same time, with the right palm facing down, arc it horizontally to the left, over the left arm, and bring both arms together in front of the abdomen. Eyes look ahead. (Figure 107)

动作十二：上动不停，左臂内旋，左掌按于左大腿根部，掌背向外，指尖斜向下，同时，上体前俯，右臂内旋，右掌前伸反手抓握左脚掌；目视左脚。（图108）

Movement 12: Without a pause, rotate the left arm inward and place the palm on the root of the left thigh, the back of palm facing out, fingers pointing diagonally downward. At the same time, bend your upper body forward and rotate the right arm inward, reaching the right palm forward to grasp the left sole. Eyes look at the left foot. (Figure 108)

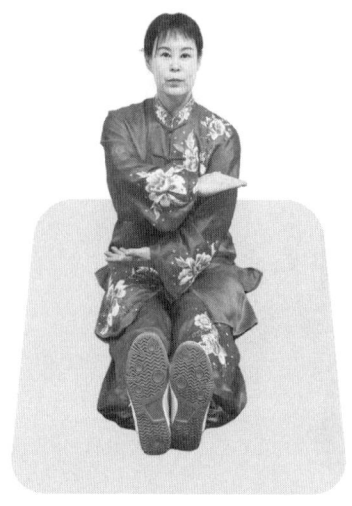
图 107/Figure 107

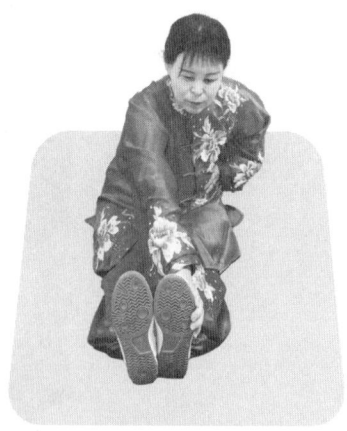
图 108/Figure 108

动作十三：上体立起，右腿膝关节稍屈，同时左腿屈膝，右手搬左脚置于右大腿下方，左手不动；目视左脚。（图 109）

Movement 13: Straighten your upper body and bend the right knee slightly. At the same time, bend the left knee, and place the left foot under the right thigh with the right hand, left hand still. Eyes look at the left foot. (Figure 109)

动作十四：右臂外旋，右掌心朝上向左画弧，同时，左掌从右臂上方向右平行画弧，两臂合于腹前；目视前方。（图 110）

Movement 14: Rotate the right arm outward, turning the palm up, then arc it horizontally to the left. At the same time, with the left palm facing down, arc it horizontally to the right, over the right arm, and bring both arms together in front of the abdomen. Eyes look ahead. (Figure 110)

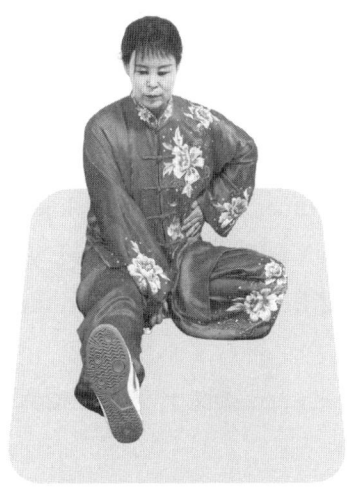 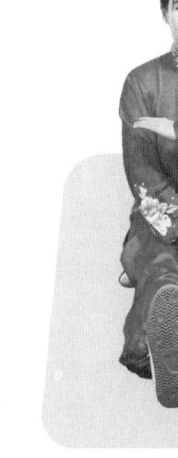

图 109/Figure 109　　　　图 110/Figure 110

动作十五：上动不停，右臂内旋，右掌按于右大腿根部，掌背向外，指尖斜向下，同时，上体前俯，左臂内旋，左掌前伸反手抓握右脚掌；目视右脚。（图 111）

Movement 15: Without a pause, rotate the right arm inward and place the palm on the root of the right thigh, the back of palm facing out, fingers pointing diagonally downward. At the same time, bend your upper body forward and rotate the left arm inward, reaching the left palm forward to grasp the right sole. Eyes look at the right foot. (Figure 111)

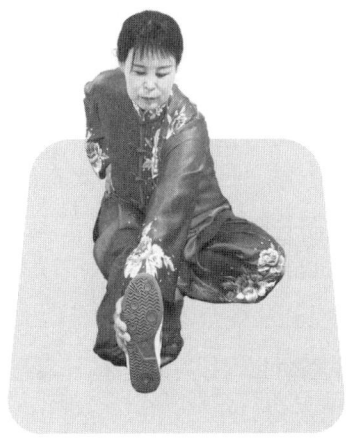

图 111/Figure 111

动作十六：上动不停，上体立起，左膝稍向上抬，同时，右腿屈膝，左手搬握右脚经左膝外侧置于左大腿下方，右手不动；目视左下方。（图112）

Movement 16: Without a pause, straighten your upper body and lift the left knee slightly. At the same time, bend the right knee, and place the right foot under the left thigh with the right hand, via the outside of the left knee, right hand still. Eyes look down to the left. (Figure 112)

动作十七：上动不停，正身端坐，左掌收于左大腿根部；目视前方。（图113）

Movement 17: Without a pause, sit up straight. Bring the left palm to rest on the root of the left thigh. Eyes look ahead. (Figure 113)

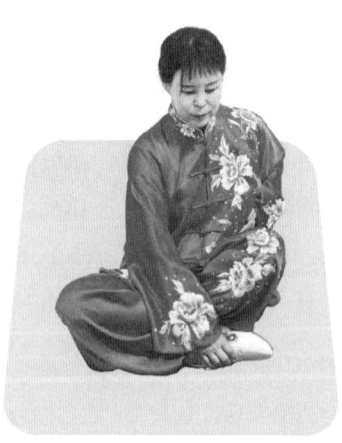
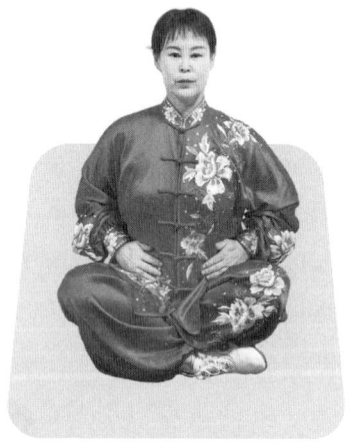

图112/Figure 112　　　　　　图113/Figure 113

二、学练要领
II. Key Points

1. 两手抓握两脚掌时，抬头、挺胸、塌腰、膝关节伸直，脚尖勾紧，要同时完成。

When grasping the soles of feet with the hands, raise your head, hold the chest up, push the waist forward, straighten the knees, and hook the toes up at the same time.

2. 抬头时，下颏主动向上用劲；下颏内收时，颈部向上伸展。

When raising your head, use the chin to push upward. When tucking the chin in, crane the neck upward.

3. 做头部动作时，两腿与腰脊要保持充分的抻拉状态。

When raising your head or tucking the chin, maintain full stretch of the legs and waist.

三、功理功用
III. Functions and Effects

1. 本式动作可刺激任脉、督脉、带脉等多条经络。可锻炼脊柱和腰背部肌肉。

This posture can stimulate the *Ren*, *Du*, and Belt meridians. It can also exercise the spine and back muscles.

2. 现代医学认为锻炼腰脊可以刺激脊髓神经和植物神经，对改善脑疾和开发大脑智力有一定作用。

Modern medicine believes that exercising the waist and spine can stimulate the spinal cord nerves and autonomic nerves, which can have a certain effect on enhancing brain health and developing intelligence.

3. 双腿伸直平坐勾脚尖能伸展马尾神经，可缓解肌肉疼痛。

Straightening the legs and sitting flat while hooking the toes up can extend the sciatic nerve, which can alleviate muscle pain.

四、适宜症状
IV. Indications

1. 有利于肾虚、糖尿病的预防和调治。

It can help to prevent and treat kidney deficiency and diabetes.

2. 可缓解神经功能紊乱所引起的不同病症。

It can alleviate the symptoms caused by neurological disorders.

3. 有利于腰背部肌肉疼痛的康复。

It is an aid to recovery from lumbar muscle pain.

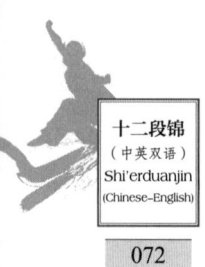

第八式　背摩精门
Posture 8　Massage Essence Gates

一、功法操作
I. Instructions

动作一：接上式，上体前俯，两掌后伸，掌心向上；目视前下方。（图 114）

Movement 1: Continuing from the end of the previous posture, bend your upper body forward and extend both hands backward, palms facing up. Eyes look down to the front. (Figure 114)

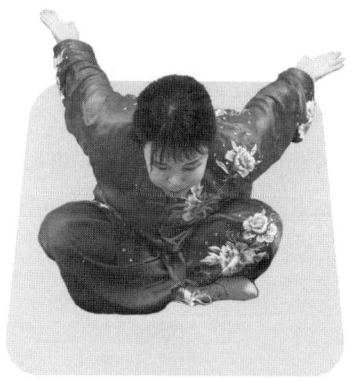

图 114/Figure 114

动作二：上动不停，两掌向体侧平摆，掌心向上；目视前下方。（图 115）

Movement 2: Without a pause, swing both hands laterally to the sides of your body, palms facing up. Eyes look down to the front. (Figure 115)

动作三：上动不停，上体立起，同时，两臂外旋，两掌弧形前摆至前平举，掌心向下；目视前方。（图 116）

Movement 3: Without a pause, straighten your upper body. At the same time, with both arms rotating outward, arc both palms forward to form a front horizontal extension, facing down. Eyes look ahead. (Figure 116)

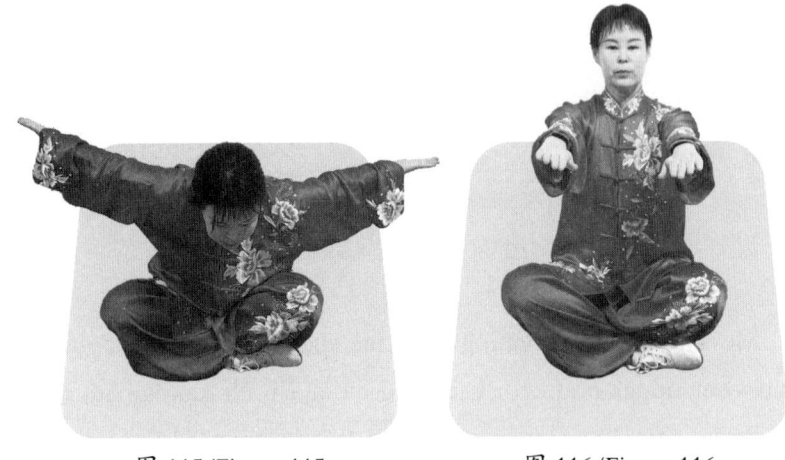

图 115/Figure 115 图 116/Figure 116

动作四：上动不停，两臂屈肘合掌于胸前，指尖向上；目视前下方。（图 117）

Movement 4: Without a pause, bend both arms to bring the palms together in front of the chest, fingers pointing up. Eyes look down to the front. (Figure 117)

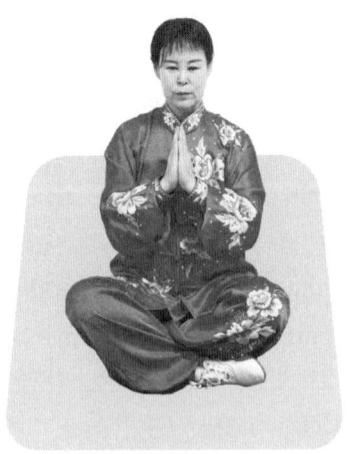

图 117/Figure 117

动作五：上动不停，两掌合紧，拧翻落于腹前，左手在上；目视前下方。（图118）

Movement 5: Without a pause, press both hands tightly together, twist and lower them down to the front of the abdomen, left hand on top. Eyes look down to the front. (Figure 118)

动作六：上动不停，两掌合紧，稍向上抬起，继续拧翻落于腹前，右手在上；目视前下方。（图119）

Movement 6: Without a pause, press both hands tightly together, lift them slightly up, then twist and lower them down to the front of the abdomen, right hand on top. Eyes look down to the front. (Figure 119)

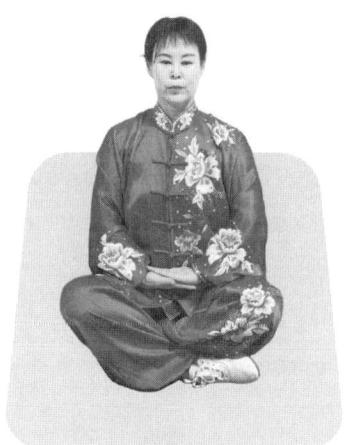
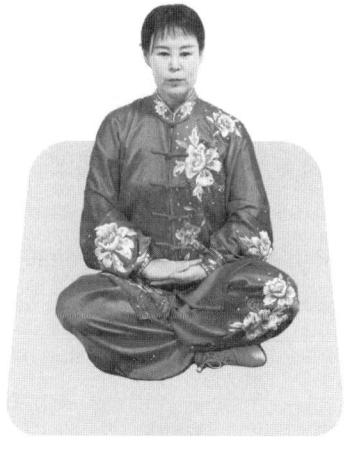

图118/Figure 118　　　　图119/Figure 119

重复动作五和动作六，左右手上下拧转翻落，共做9遍。第9遍左手在上。接做动作七。

Repeat Movements 5 and 6. Lift both hands up, twist and lower them down for a total of nine times. For the ninth repetition, left hand is on top. Do Movement 7.

动作七：上体保持中正，左臂外旋，右臂内旋，两手贴腹部两侧；目视前下方。（图120）

Movement 7: With your upper body upright, rotate the left arm outward and the right arm inward, palms placed against the sides of the abdomen. Eyes look down to the front. (Figure 120)

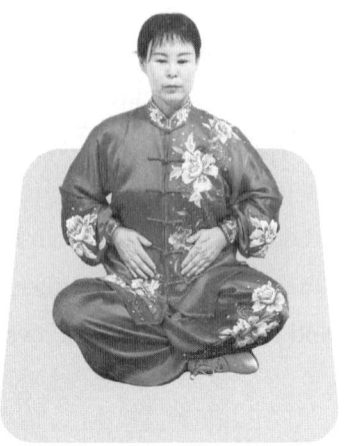

图 120/Figure 120

动作八：身体姿势保持不变，两手向后摩运至后腰处的肾俞穴，转掌指向斜下；目视前下方。（图 121 正面、图 121 背面）

Movement 8: With the position of your upper body unchanged, rub both hands backward to the *Shenshu* acupoints on both sides of the lower back. Rotate the palms to face diagonally downward. Eyes look down to the front. (Figure 121 front, Figure 121 back)

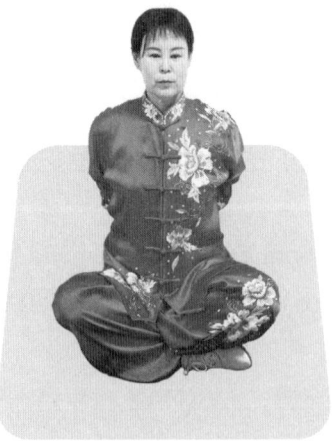 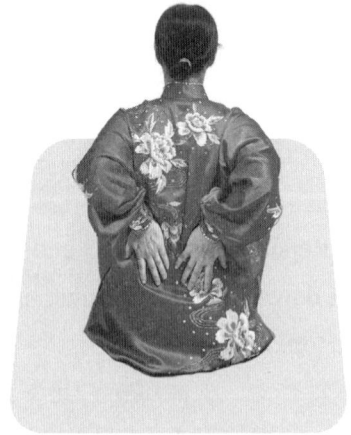

图 121 正面 /Figure 121 front   图 121 背面 /Figure 121 back

动作九：身体姿势保持不变，两掌贴后腰部稍用力，向下按摩至臀部；目视前方。（图 122 正面、图 122 背面）

Movement 9: Maintain the position of your upper body unchanged. With slightly more pressure, massage from the lower back downward to the buttocks with both palms. Eyes look ahead. (Figure 122 front, Figure 122 back)

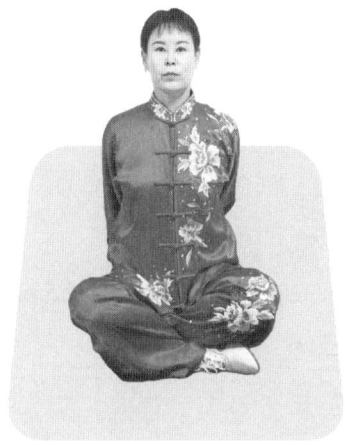 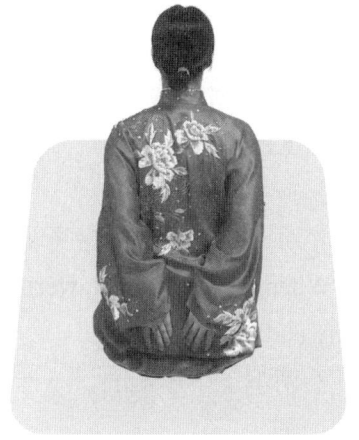

图 122 正面 /Figure 122 front   图 122 背面 /Figure 122 back

动作十：身体姿势保持不变，两掌轻贴身体从臀部向上摩运至后腰处的肾俞穴；目视前下方。（图 123）

Movement 10: Maintain the position of your upper body

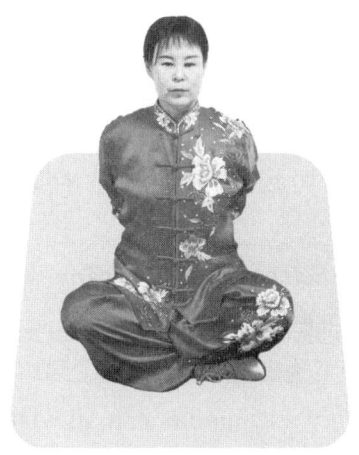

图 123/Figure 123

unchanged. Massage lightly with both hands from the buttocks upward to *Shenshu* acupoints at the lower back. Eyes look down to the front. (Figure 123)

重复动作九和动作十，一下一上为1遍，上下连续摩擦共做24遍。

Repeat Movements 9 and 10. Massaging downward and upward form a round. Do twenty-four rounds.

二、学练要领
II. Key Points

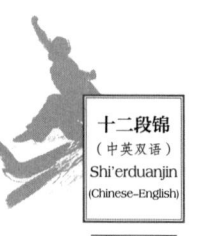

1. 两掌合拢做拧转翻落动作时，掌心要压紧搓热。

When twisting and lowering the clasped hands, press the palms tightly and rub them hot.

2. 两掌上下摩运时，五指并拢，掌心含空，上轻下重，速度适中。

When massaging upward or downward with both hands, the fingers should be closed together, palms hollow. Apply less force when massaging upward, and more force when massaging downward, with a moderate speed.

三、功理功用
III. Functions and Effects

1. 摩擦肾俞穴，可起到温通经络，补肾益气，强壮腰肌的作用。

Massaging *Shenshu* acupoints can warm the meridians, regulate the kidneys, nourish *Qi*, and strengthen the waist muscle.

2. 按摩劳宫穴可以缓解烦闷、焦虑、易怒等情绪。

Massaging *Laogong* acupoints can alleviate emotions such as anxiety, irritability, and restlessness.

四、适宜症状
IV. Indications

有预防和缓解腰痛、下肢无力、阳痿、痛经等效果。

It can prevent and relieve symptoms such as lower back pain, leg weakness, impotence, and menstrual pain.

第九式 前抚脘腹

Posture 9 Caress Upper and Lower Abdomen

一、功法操作
I. Instructions

动作一：接上式，身体保持中正，两掌稍向上提至腰两侧，指尖斜向下；目视前方。（图 124）

Movement 1: Continuing from the end of the previous posture, with your upper body upright, lift both palms slightly upward to the sides of the waist, fingers pointing diagonally down. Eyes look ahead. (Figure 124)

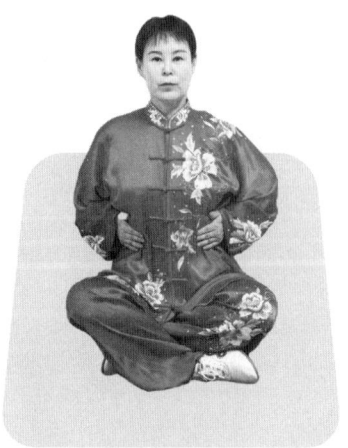

图 124/Figure 124

动作二：上动不停，两掌贴肋转掌指向前，两指尖斜相对；目视前方。（图 125）

Movement 2: Without a pause, rotate the palms against the ribs to point forward, fingers pointing each other diagonally. Eyes look ahead. (Figure 125)

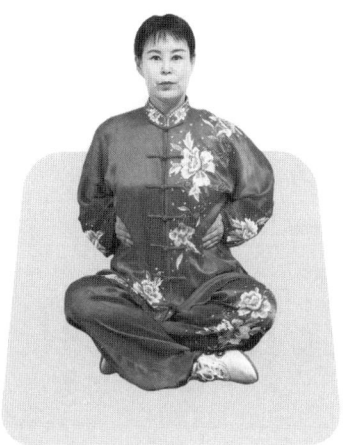

图 125/Figure 125

动作三：上动不停，两掌贴肋向前横向摩运至乳下，指尖相对；目视前方。（图 126）

Movement 3: Without a pause, rub both palms forward against the ribs horizontally to the lower part of the chest, fingers pointing each other. Eyes look ahead. (Figure 126)

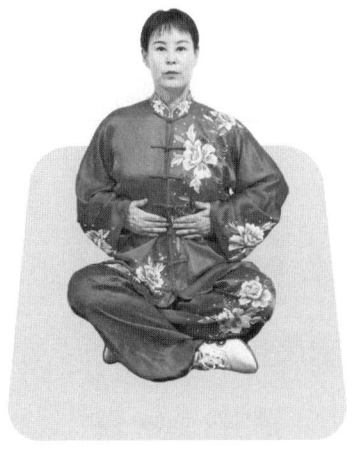

图 126/Figure 126

动作四：上动不停，两掌贴肋转指尖向下；目视前方。（图 127）

Movement 4: Without a pause, rotate the palms against the ribs to point down. Eyes look ahead. (Figure 127)

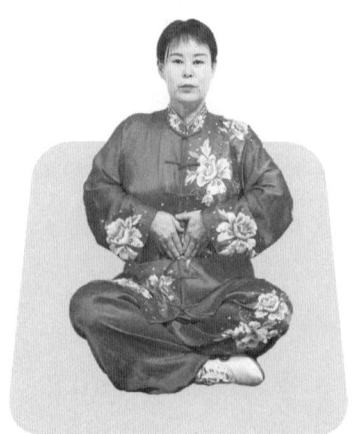

图 127/Figure 127

动作五：上动不停，两掌贴肋顺腹前向下摩运至下腹部；目视前方。（图 128）

Movement 5: Without a pause, rub both palms downward against the ribs along the front of the abdomen to the lower abdomen. Eyes look ahead. (Figure 128)

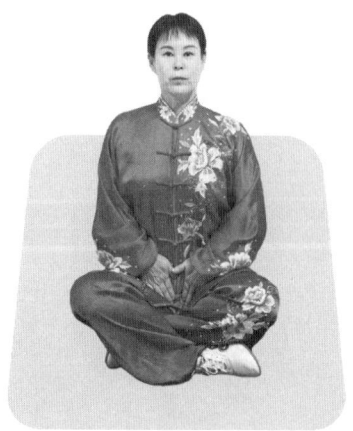

图 128/Figure 128

动作六：上动不停，身体保持中正，两掌转指尖斜相对；目视前方。（图 129）

Movement 6: Without a pause, maintain your upper body upright. Rotate the fingers to point each other diagonally. Eyes look ahead. (Figure 129)

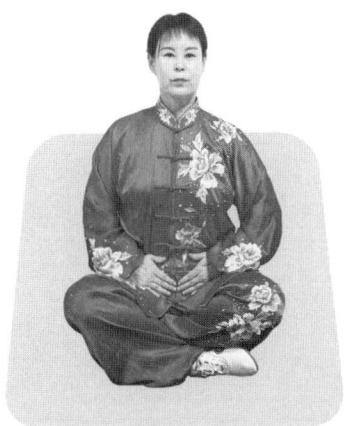

图 129/Figure 129

动作七：上动不停，两掌向两侧摩运，指尖斜相对；目视前方。（图 130）

Movement 7: Without a pause, rub both hands to the sides of the abdomen, fingers pointing each other diagonally. Eyes look ahead. (Figure 130)

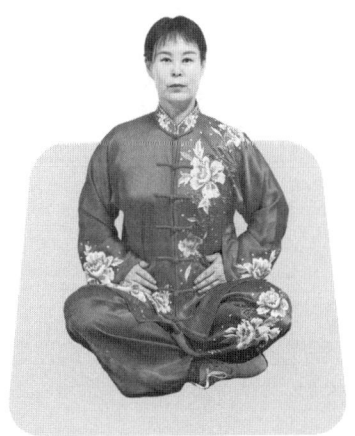

图 130/Figure 130

动作八：上动不停，身体保持中正，两掌转指尖斜向下；目视前方。（图 131）

Movement 8: Without a pause, maintain your upper body upright. Rotate the fingers to point diagonally down. Eyes look ahead. (Figure 131)

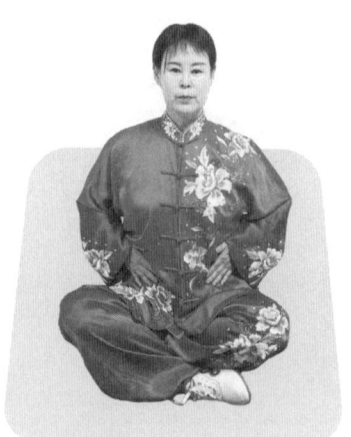

图 131/Figure 131

动作九：上动不停，两掌沿胁肋部向上摩运至两乳下，指尖斜向下；目视前方。（图 132）

Movement 9: Without a pause, rub both palms upward against the ribs to the lower part of the chest, fingers pointing diagonally down. Eyes look ahead. (Figure 132)

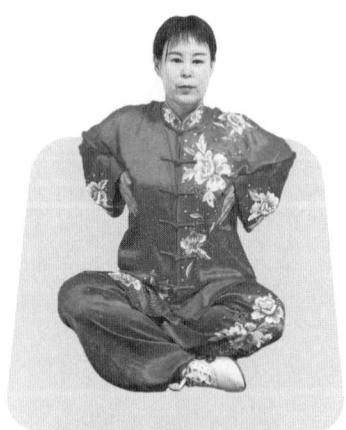

图 132/Figure 132

重复动作二至动作九，一下一上为 1 遍，共做 6 遍。第 6 遍结束时，接做动作十。

Repeat Movements 2 through 9. Rubbing both palms down and up forms a round. Do six rounds. After the sixth round, do Movement 10.

动作十：上动不停，两掌贴肋转掌指向前，两指尖斜相对；目视前方。（图 133）

Movement 10: Without a pause, rotate the palms against the ribs to point forward, fingers pointing each other diagonally. Eyes look ahead. (Figure 133)

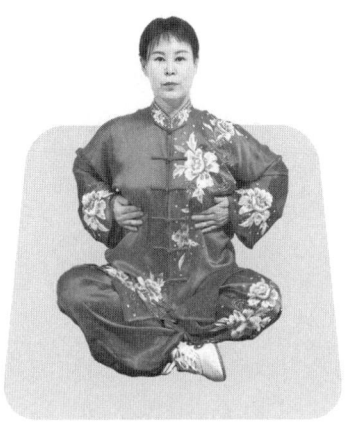

图 133/Figure 133

动作十一：上动不停，两掌贴肋向前横向摩运至乳下，指尖相对；目视前方。（图 134）

Movement 11: Without a pause, rub both palms forward against the ribs horizontally to the lower part of the chest, fingers pointing each other. Eyes look ahead. (Figure 134)

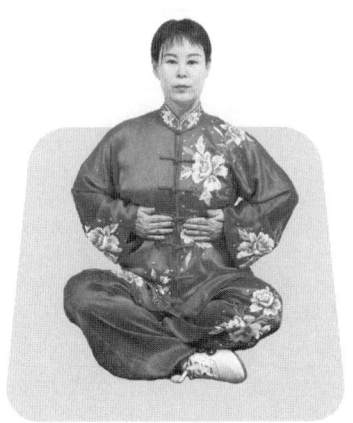

图 134/Figure 134

动作十二：上动不停，两掌贴肋转指尖向下；目视前方。（图135）

Movement 12: Without a pause, rotate the palms against the ribs to point downward. Eyes look ahead. (Figure 135)

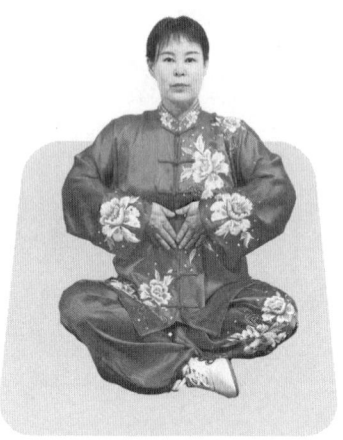

图 135/Figure 135

动作十三：上动不停，两掌贴肋顺腹前向下摩运至下腹部；目视前方。（图136）

Movement 13: Without a pause, rub both palms downward against the ribs along the front of the abdomen to the lower abdomen. Eyes look ahead. (Figure 136)

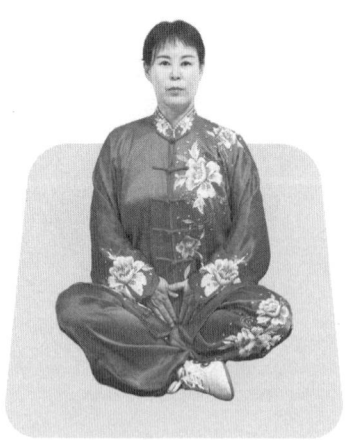

图 136/Figure 136

动作十四：上动不停，两掌经下腹部向上摩运至两乳下，指尖斜向下；目视前方。（图 137）

Movement 14: Without a pause, rub both palms upward against the ribs to the lower part of the chest, fingers pointing diagonally down. Eyes look ahead. (Figure 137)

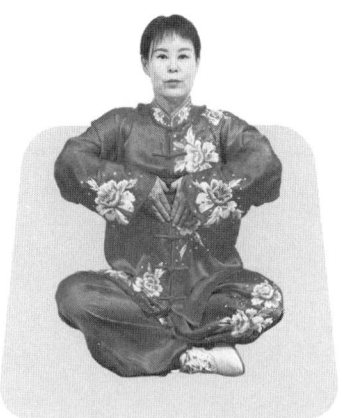

图 137/Figure 137

动作十五：上动不停，身体保持中正，两掌贴肋转指尖相对；目视前方。（图 138）

Movement 15: Without a pause, maintain your upper body upright. Rotate the hands against the ribs to point each other. Eyes look ahead. (Figure 138)

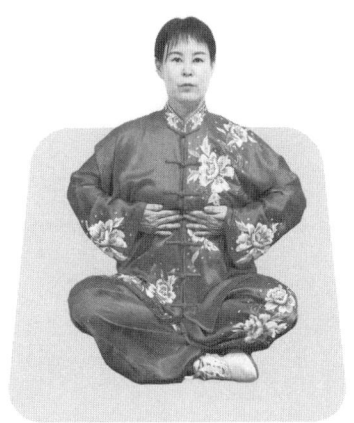

图 138/Figure 138

动作十六：上动不停，两掌向身体左右两侧横向摩运，指尖相对；目视前方。（图 139）

Movement 16: Without a pause, rub both palms against the ribs horizontally to the sides of your body, fingers pointing each other. Eyes look ahead. (Figure 139)

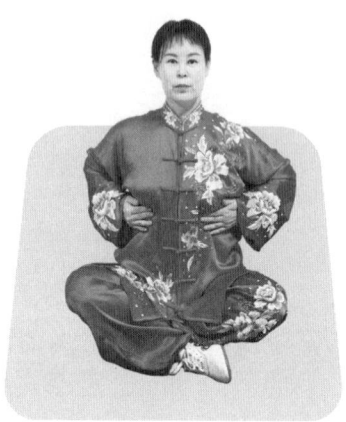

图 139/Figure 139

动作十七：上动不停，两掌由上向下沿两胁肋部摩运至下腹部，指尖斜相对；目视前方。（图 140）

Movement 17: Without a pause, rub both palms from the upper to the lower abdomen along the rib cage, fingers pointing each other diagonally. Eyes look ahead. (Figure 140)

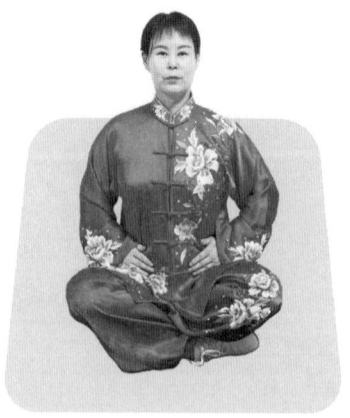

图 140/Figure 140

动作十八：上动不停，身体保持中正，两掌从腹部左右两侧向内横向摩运，指尖相对；目视前方。（图 141）

Movement 18: Without a pause, maintain your upper body upright. Rub both palms horizontally inward from both sides of the abdomen, fingers pointing each other. Eyes look ahead. (Figure 141)

动作十九：上动不停，两掌贴腹部转指尖向下；目视前方。（图 142）

Movement 19: Without a pause, rotate both palms against the abdomen to point downward. Eyes look ahead. (Figure 142)

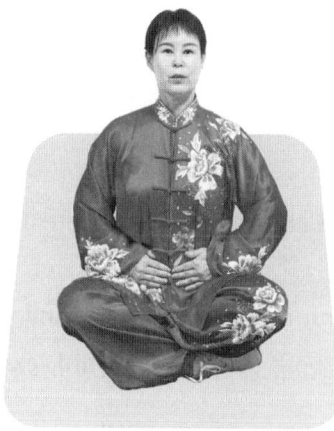
图 141/Figure 141

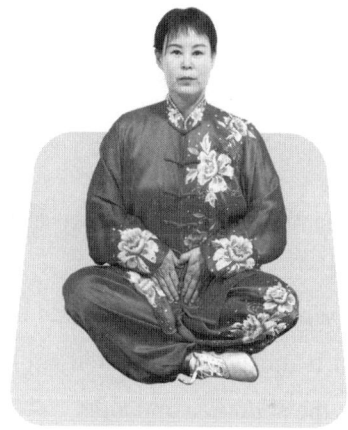
图 142/Figure 142

重复动作十四至动作十九，一上一下为 1 遍，共做 6 遍。

Repeat Movements 14 through 19. Rubbing both palms upward and downward forms a round. Do six rounds.

第 6 遍时，两掌由上向下摩运至两胁肋部，指尖斜相对；目视前方。（图 143）

On the sixth round, rub both palms downward to the rib cage, fingers pointing each other diagonally. Eyes look ahead. (Figure 143)

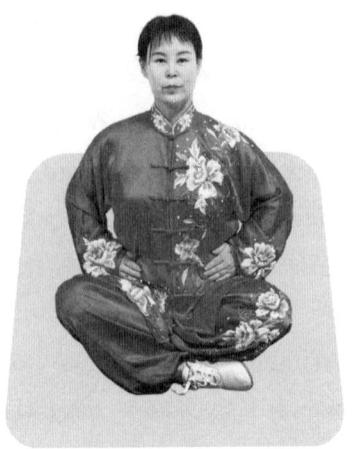

图 143/Figure 143

二、学练要领
II. Key Points

1. 向上摩运时，吸气、收腹、提肛；向下摩运时，呼气、松腹、松肛。

When rubbing both palms upward, inhale, contract the abdomen, and lift up the anus. When rubbing both palms downward, exhale, relax the abdomen and anus.

2. 两掌上下摩运时速度要均匀，用力要适度。

When rubbing both palms up or down, keep the pace even and apply moderate force.

三、功理功用
III. Functions and Effects

1. 通过对腹部的按摩，可调和气血，疏通经络，促进腹腔脏器的血液循环。

Massaging the abdomen can help to regulate the circulation of *Qi* and blood, and unblock meridians, promoting the blood circulation of abdominal organs.

2. 疏肝理气，调理脾胃，改善消化、泌尿生殖系统功能。

It can help to soothe the liver and regulate *Qi*, improve digestion, and enhance the functions of the digestive and urogenital systems.

四、适宜症状
IV. Indications

可以预防和缓解腹部胀满不适、便秘、高血压、糖尿病、脂肪肝、失眠等症状。

It can prevent and alleviate symptoms such as abdominal fullness and discomfort, constipation, hypertension, diabetes, fatty liver, and insomnia.

第十式　温煦脐轮

Posture 10　Warm Navel Ring

一、功法操作
I. Instructions

动作一：接上式，身体中正，两掌相对横向摩运，叠于肚脐处，左掌在里轻抚肚脐，右掌在外轻抚左掌；两眼垂帘。（图144）

Movement 1: Continuing from the end of the previous posture, with your upper body upright, rub your palms together horizontally to overlap them at the navel. The left palm is inside, lightly caressing the navel; while the right palm is outside, lightly caressing the left palm. Close your eyes lightly. (Figure 144)

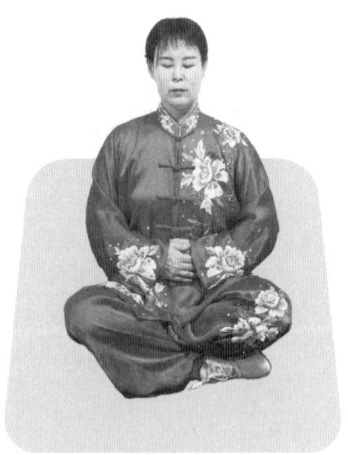

图 144/Figure 144

动作二：两眼睁开，两掌顺时针摩腹3周；目视前下方。（图145）

Movement 2: Open your eyes. Massage your abdomen with the palms clockwise for three circles. Eyes look down to the front. (Figure 145)

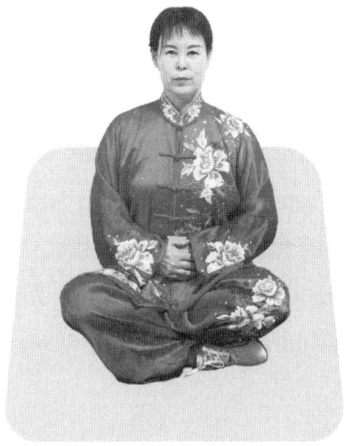

图 145/Figure 145

动作三：身体姿势保持不变，逆时针摩腹 3 周；目视前下方。（图 146）

Movement 3: With the position of your upper body unchanged, massage your abdomen counterclockwise for three circles. Eyes look down to the front. (Figure 146)

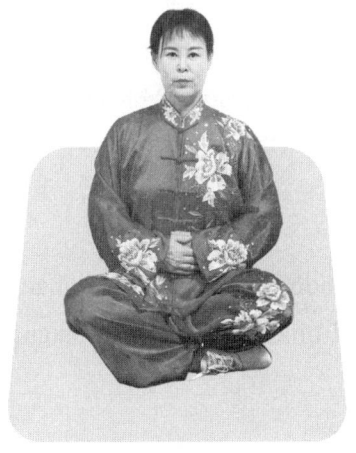

图 146/Figure 146

二、学练要领
II. Key Points

1. 两眼垂帘时，意想脐轮有温热感，用意要轻，身体保持中正安舒，约3至5分钟。

When the eyes are closed, imagine that there is a warm sensation around the navel ring. Use your mind lightly and maintain your upper body upright and comfortable for about 3 to 5 minutes.

2. 揉按腹部时，劳宫对准肚脐，柔和缓慢，呼吸自然。

When massaging the abdomen, point *Laogong* acupoints to the navel and massage in a gentle and slow manner while breathing naturally.

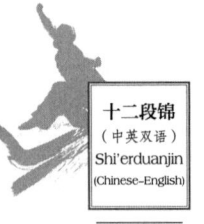

三、功理功用
III. Functions and Effects

1. 意守脐轮可养气安神、固本培元，有促进心肾相交、调节阴阳平衡的作用。

Focusing your mind on the navel ring can cultivate vital energy, calm the spirit, strengthen the root and promote the interaction between the heart and kidneys, regulating the balance of *Yin* and *Yang*.

2. 有助于舒缓交感神经的紧张状态，起到调节情绪的作用。

It helps to reduce the tension of the sympathetic nervous system, regulating emotions.

3. 揉按腹部可疏通经络、调和气血，避免由于用意过重而出现结气现象。

Massaging the abdomen can unblock channels and regulate the circulation of *Qi* and blood, avoiding *Qi* stagnation from excessive concentration.

四、适宜症状
IV. Indications

可以预防和缓解情绪紧张、失眠、腹部胀满不适、便秘、高血压等症状。

It can prevent and alleviate symptoms such as emotional stress, insomnia, abdominal fullness and discomfort, constipation, and hypertension.

第十一式 摇身晃海

Posture 11　Rotate Upper Body

一、功法操作
I. Instructions

动作一：接上式，上身姿势保持不变，两掌分开前伸，分别扶于两膝上，掌心向下；目视前方。（图 147）

Movement 1: Continuing from the end of the previous posture, with the position of your upper body unchanged, separate the hands and extend them forward, placing them on both knees, palms facing down. Eyes look ahead. (Figure 147)

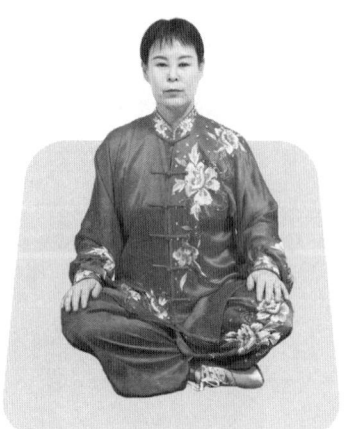

图 147/Figure 147

动作二：上体稍左倾，身体保持斜中寓正，两手扶于两膝上；两眼垂帘。（图 148）

Movement 2: Tilt your upper body slightly to the left, with a diagonal balance, palms on knees. Close your eyes lightly. (Figure 148)

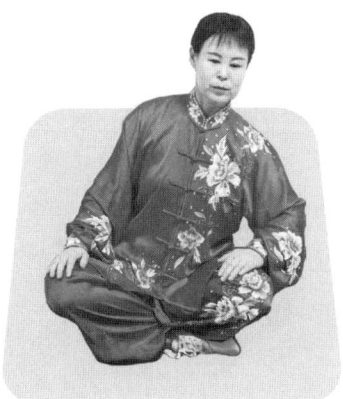

图 148/Figure 148

动作三：上动不停，上体从左向前绕环至稍前倾，微低头、含胸、松腰，两手扶于两膝上；两眼垂帘。（图 149）

Movement 3: Without a pause, rotate your upper body from the left to the front until it leans slightly forward, head slightly lowered, chest drawn in, waist relaxed, hands on knees. Close your eyes lightly. (Figure 149)

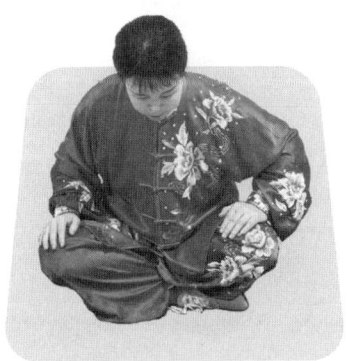

图 149/Figure 149

动作四：上动不停，上体从前向右绕环至稍右倾，身体保持斜中寓正，两手扶于两膝上；两眼垂帘。（图 150）

Movement 4: Without a pause, rotate your upper body from the front to the right, with a diagonal balance, palms on knees. Close your eyes lightly. (Figure 150)

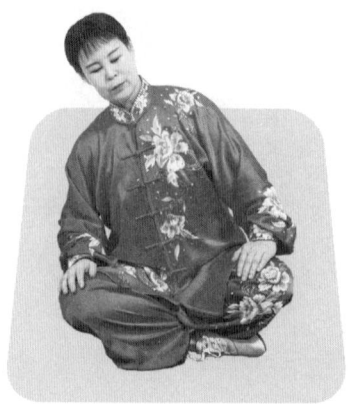

图 150/Figure 150

动作五：上动不停，上体从右向左绕至立身端坐，两手扶于两膝上；两眼垂帘。（图 151）

Movement 5: Without a pause, rotate your upper body from the right to the left until you sit erect, palms on knees. Close your eyes lightly. (Figure 151)

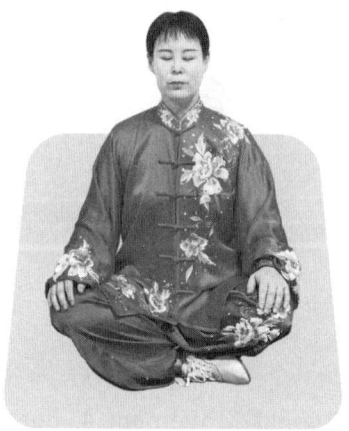

图 151/Figure 151

动作二至动作五，顺时针绕转共 6 圈。

Repeat Movements 2 throgh 5 clockwise six times.

动作六：同动作二，唯左右相反。（图 152）

Movement 6: Repeat Movement 2, but with left and right reversed. (Figure 152)

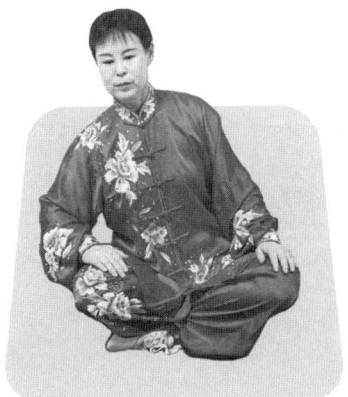

图 152/Figure 152

动作七：同动作三，唯左右相反。（图 153）

Movement 7: Repeat Movement 3, but with left and right reversed. (Figure 153)

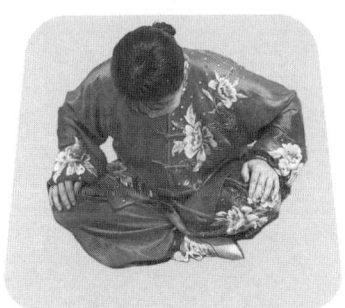

图 153/Figure 153

动作八：同动作四，唯左右相反。（图 154）

Movement 8: Repeat Movement 4, but with left and right reversed. (Figure 154)

动作九：同动作五，唯左右相反。（图 155）

Movement 9: Repeat Movement 5, but with left and right reversed. (Figure 155)

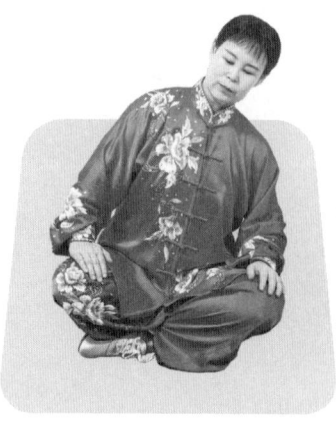
图 154/Figure 154

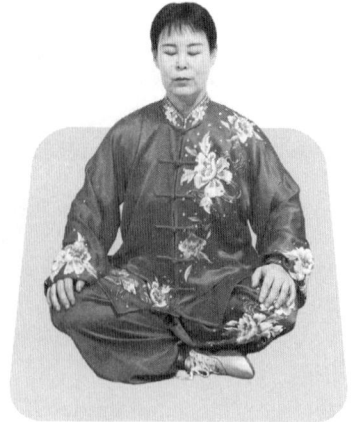
图 155/Figure 155

动作六至动作九,逆时针绕转共 6 圈。

Repeat Movements 6 through 9 counterclockwise six times.

动作十:两眼睁开,正身端坐;目视前方。(图 156)

Movement 10: Open your eyes, and sit up straight. Eyes look ahead. (Figure 156)

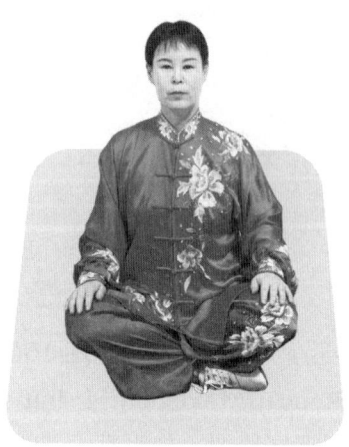
图 156/Figure 156

二、学练要领
II. Key Points

1. 上体绕转时,要百会虚领,下颏微收,立项竖脊。运动速度要均匀，圆活连贯。

When rotating your upper body, pull up *Baihui* acupoint, chin slightly tucked in, spine erect. The movements should be smooth and consistent, with an even speed.

2. 幅度不宜过大，两膝不要抬起，保持稳定。

The range of rotation should not be too large. Don't lift the knees. Keep steady.

3. 内视海底，引气归元。

Visualize *Haidi* and guide *Qi* back to its origin.

三、功理功用
III. Functions and Effects

1. 内视海底，可畅通任督二脉，调和气血，引气归元。

Visualizing *Haidi* can smooth the *Ren* and *Du* meridians, regulate *Qi* and blood circulation and guide *Qi* back to its origin.

2. 摇晃脊柱可强壮腰脊，对腹腔脏器有良好的按摩作用，可刺激其活力，改善其功能。

Rotating the spinc can strengthen it at the waist and massage the abdominal organs to stimulate their vitality and improve their functions.

四、适宜症状
IV. Indications

可以预防和缓解阳痿早泄、失眠症、神经衰弱、腰酸背痛等症状。

It can prevent and alleviate symptoms such as impotence and premature ejaculation, insomnia, neurasthenia, and backache.

第十二式 鼓漱吞津
Posture 12　Gargle and Swallow

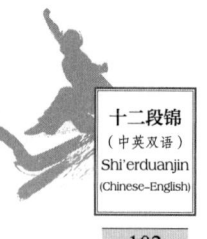

一、功法操作
I. Instructions

动作一：接上式，上身姿势保持不变，两臂内旋，两掌回收经腰间向两侧画弧，掌心向后；目视前下方。（图 157）

Movement 1: Continuing from the end of the previous posture, maintain the position of your upper body unchanged. With both arms rotating inward, bring the palms back to the waist and arc them toward both sides of your upper body, facing backward. Eyes look down to the front. (Figure 157)

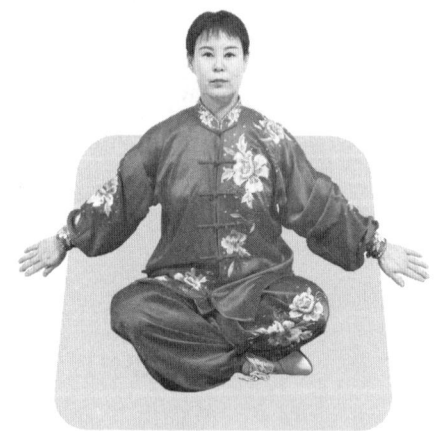

图 157/Figure 157

动作二：上动不停，两臂外旋，掌心向前；目视前下方。（图 158）

Movement 2: Without a pause, rotate both arms outward, palms facing forward. Eyes look down to the front. (Figure 158)

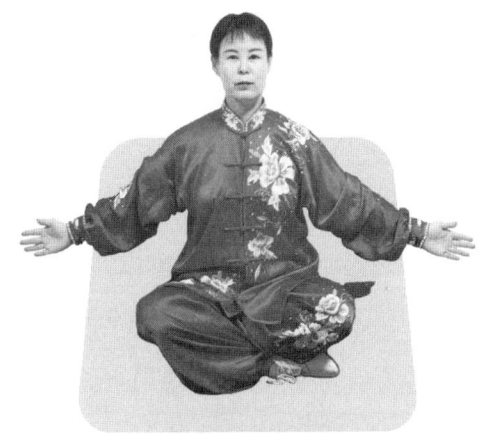

图 158/Figure 158

动作三：上动不停，两掌弧形向腹前合抱，指尖相对，与肚脐同高；目视前下方。（图 159）

Movement 3: Without a pause, bring both palms forward in an arc to the front of the abdomen, fingers pointing each other at the height of the navel. Eyes look down to the front. (Figure 159)

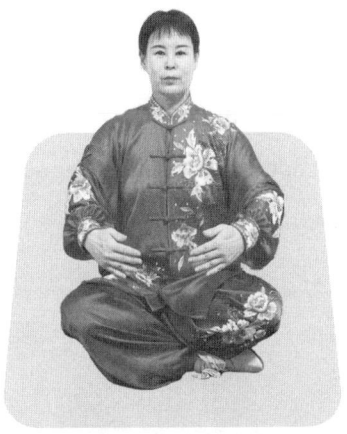

图 159/Figure 159

动作四：上动不停，屈肘两掌回收接近肚脐时握固，落于大腿根部，拳眼向上；目视前下方。（图 160）

Movement 4: Without a pause, bend the elbows and clench both palms into fists as you bring them closer to the navel, then place the fists on the roots of your thighs, the eyes of fists facing up. Eyes look down to the front. (Figure 160)

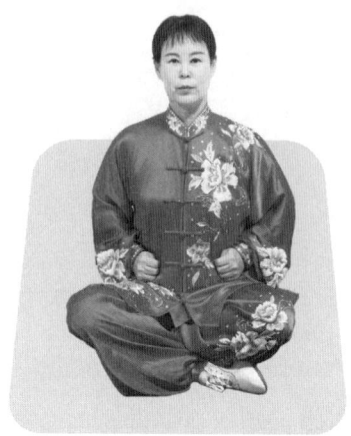

图 160/Figure 160

动作五：身体姿势保持不变，唇口轻闭，舌尖在口腔内由右向上、向左、向下绕转1圈后，舌尖移到牙齿外，贴牙龈由右向上、向左、向下绕转1圈。一内一外为1遍，共做6遍。目视前下方。（图161）

Movement 5: With the position of your upper body unchanged, close the lips lightly and arc the tongue from the right, upward, to the left, and downward inside the mouth, then move the tongue outside

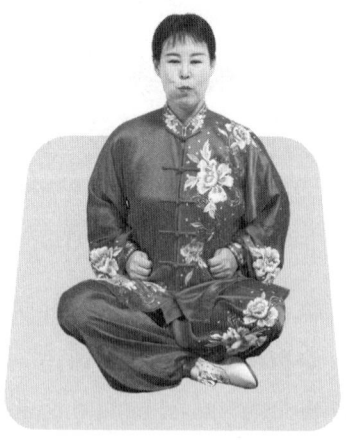

图 161/Figure 161

the teeth, arcing it from the right upward, to the left, and downward along the gum. One inner circle and one outer circle form a round. Do six rounds. Eyes look down to the front. (Figure 161)

动作六：同动作五，唯左右相反。（图 162）

Movement 6: Repeat Movement 5, but with left and right reversed. (Figure 162)

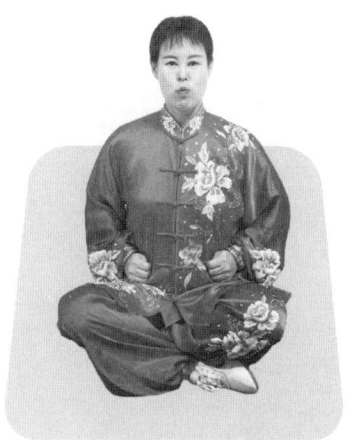

图 162/Figure 162

动作七：接上动，两腮做鼓漱 36 次；目视前下方。（图 163）

Movement 7: Continuing from the end of the previous movement, gargle with saliva thirty-six times. Eyes look down to the front. (Figure 163)

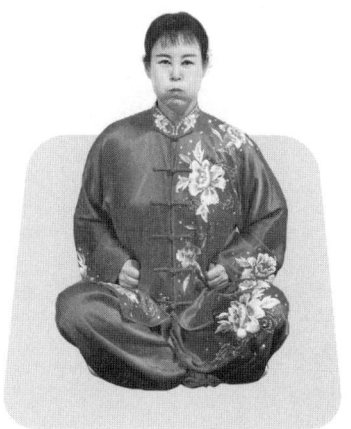

图 163/Figure 163

动作八：接上动，两臂外旋，两拳变掌上举至胸前，掌心向外；目视前下方。（图164）

Movement 8: Continuing from the end of the previous movement, with both arms rotating outward, open both fists to palms and lift them up to the chest, facing out. Eyes look down to the front. (Figure 164)

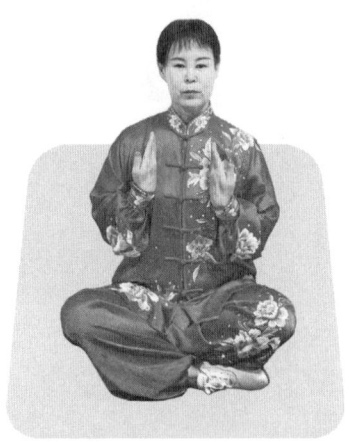

图164/Figure 164

动作九：上动不停，两臂内旋直臂上举至头上方，掌心向外；目视前方。（图165）

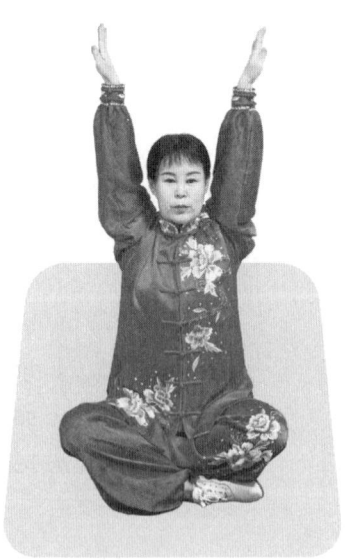

图165/Figure 165

Movement 9: Without a pause, rotate both arms inward and extend them up above your head, palms facing out. Eyes look ahead. (Figure 165)

动作十：两臂外旋，两手在头上方握固，拳心相对；目视前下方。（图 166）

Movement 10: With both arms rotating outward, clench your fists over your head, the hearts of fists facing each other. Eyes look down to the front. (Figure 166)

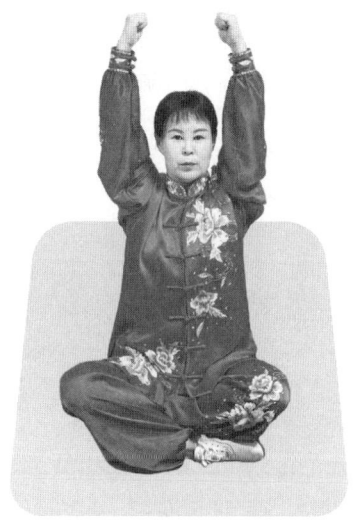

图 166/Figure 166

动作十一：上动不停，两拳下拉置于大腿根部，拳眼向上，同时，吞咽口中 1/3 的津液，用意念送至丹田；目视前下方。（图 167）

Movement 11: Without a pause, pull both fists downward to the roots of your thighs, the eyes of your fists facing up. At the same time, swallow a third of the saliva, imagining the saliva is transported to *Dantian*. Eyes look down to the front. (Figure 167)

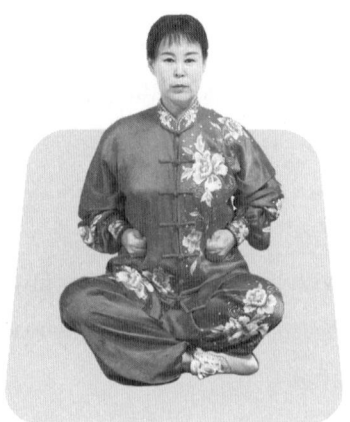

图 167/Figure 167

动作八至动作十一共做3遍，口中津液分3次咽下。

Repeat Movements 8 through 11 three times, and swallow the saliva in three times.

二、学练要领
II. Key Points

1. 在练习本式时，意念口中生满津液。

In this posture, imagine your mouth is full of saliva.

2. 舌在口中搅动时，要圆活连贯。

The tongue should move in the mouth smoothly and continuously.

3. 做鼓漱动作时，两腮要快速抖动。

When gargling, the cheeks should quickly shake.

4. 吞咽口中津液时，要发出"汩汩"响声，意送丹田。

When swallowing the saliva, make a "gurgling" sound and imagine the saliva is transported to *Dantian*.

三、功理功用
III. Functions and Effects

1. 舌的搅动与鼓漱可促进唾液分泌。唾液有杀菌、清洁口腔、防治牙龈炎和牙龈萎缩的作用。

The movement of your tongue and gargling can promote saliva secretion, which can kill bacteria, clean the mouth, prevent and treat gingivitis and gum recession.

2. 吞津可调节全身气息，灌溉五脏，营养周身，有消食化瘀、解除疲劳、延缓衰老、增进健康的作用。

Swallowing saliva can regulate Qi, tone the internal organs, nourish the whole body, help digestion, remove extravasated blood, relieve fatigue, delay aging, and improve health.

四、适宜症状
IV. Indications

可以预防和缓解腰膝酸软、遗精漏尿、阳痿早泄等症状。

It can prevent and alleviate symptoms such as soreness of the lower back and knees, nocturnal emission, enuresis, impotence and premature ejaculation.

收 势
Closing

一、功法操作
I. Instructions

动作一：接上式，两拳经腰间向前伸，左臂在内，两腕在胸前交叉，拳心向内，稍用力前撑，同时胸部微含，背向后倚，动作略停；目视前方。（图 168）

Movement 1: Continuing from the end of the previous posture, extend both fists forward from the waist and cross the wrists in front of the chest, with the left arm inside, the hearts of your fists facing inward. Apply a slight force forward in the fists while leaning backward with your back, chest drawn in. Pause for a while. Eyes look ahead. (Figure 168)

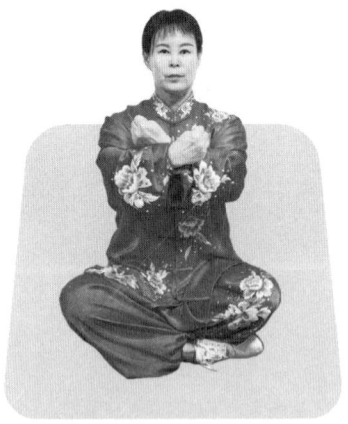

图 168/Figure 168

动作二：两拳变掌下落置于膝上，掌心向上；目视前方。（图169）

Movement 2: Open both fists into palms and lower them to rest on the knees, palms facing up. Eyes look ahead. (Figure 169)

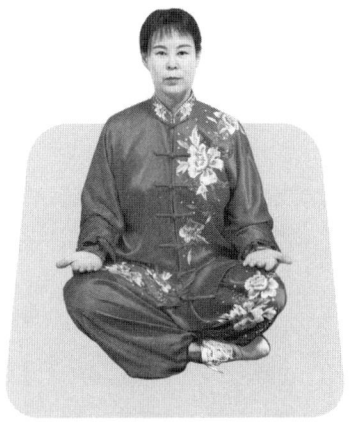

图 169/Figure 169

动作三：两掌从膝上两侧弧形向体前斜上方托起，肘关节微屈；目视前上方。（图 170）

Movement 3: Lift both palms upward in an arc from the knees to the diagonal upper fronts of your body respectively, elbows slightly bent. Eyes look up to the front. (Figure 170)

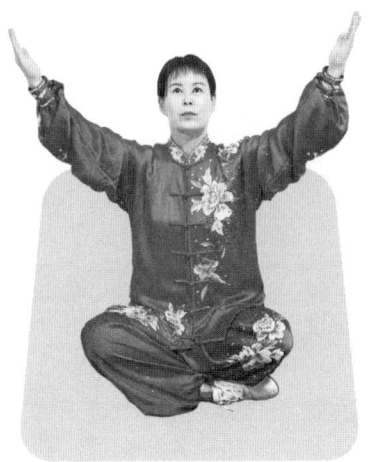

图 170/Figure 170

动作四：身体保持中正，下颌内收，两臂内旋，两掌下落至前平举，与肩同宽，掌心向下；目视前方。（图 171）

Movement 4: With your body upright, tuck in the chin and rotate both arms inward, lowering both palms to a horizontal position in front of your body, shoulder-width apart, facing down. Eyes look ahead. (Figure 171)

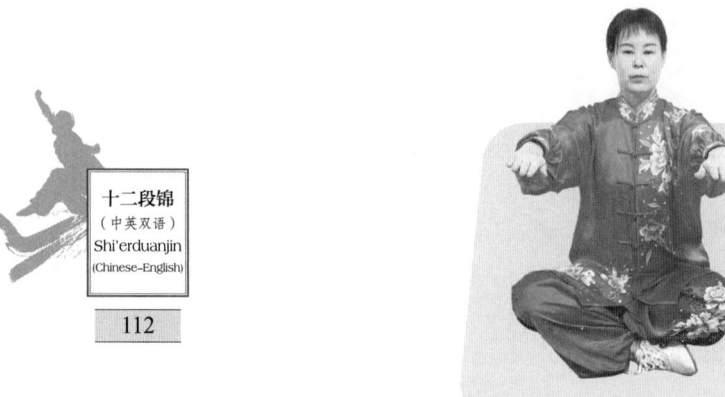

图 171/Figure 171

动作五：上动不停，两掌由身前下按，扶于膝关节内侧，略停；目视前方。（图 172）

Movement 5: Without a pause, press both palms downward in front of your body to rest them on the inner knees. Pause for a while.

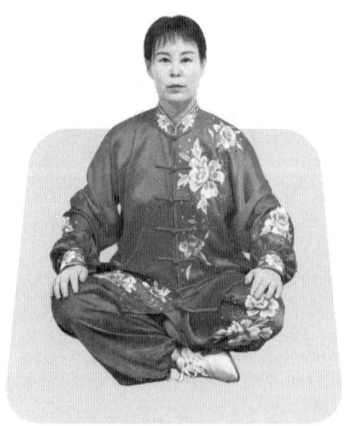

图 172/Figure 172

Eyes look ahead. (Figure 172)

动作六：两掌沿大腿外侧下落至十指撑地；目视前下方。（图173）

Movement 6: Lower both palms along the outer thighs to rest them on the ground with ten fingers. Eyes look down to the front. (Figure 173)

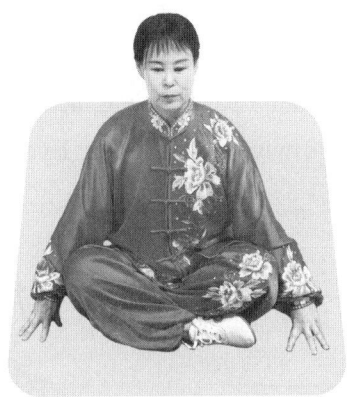

图 173/Figure 173

动作七：上动不停，上体前俯，同时十指与两脚撑地；目视前下方。（图 174）

Movement 7: Without a pause, lean your upper body forward. At the same time, support your body on ten fingers and both feet. Eyes look down to the front. (Figure 174)

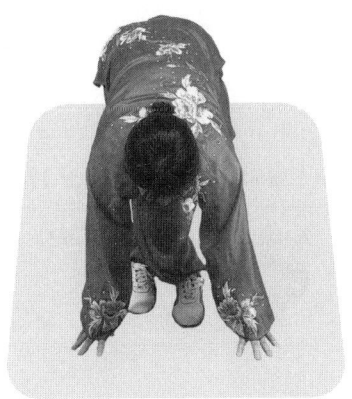

图 174/Figure 174

动作八：上动不停，顺势身体向上立起，随之右脚向右斜前方上步，两掌垂于体侧；目视前方。（图175）

Movement 8: Without a pause, stand up with the momentum and take a step forward with the right foot to the right. Allow both palms to hang down on both sides of your body. Eyes look ahead. (Figure 175)

动作九：上动不停，左脚收于右脚内侧成并步站立；目视前方。（图176）

Movement 9: Without a pause, bring the left foot to the inside of the right foot and stand with feet together. Eyes look ahead. (Figure 176)

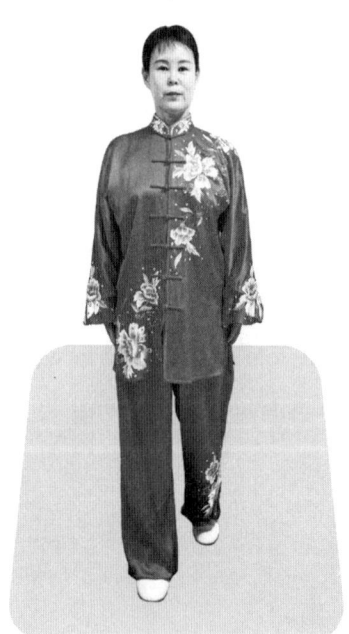
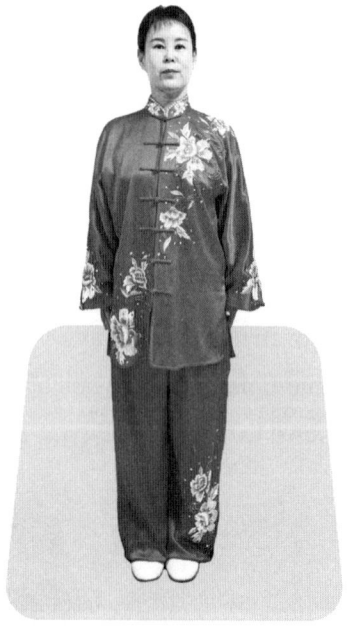

图 175/Figure 175　　　　图 176/Figure 176

二、学练要领
II. Key Points

1. 两腕在胸前交叉时，拳要握紧，咬牙，闭气。

When crossing both wrists in front of the chest, clench the fists and teeth tightly, and hold breath.

2. 两手由拳变掌下落时，意想周身放松、气血通畅。

When opening the fists into palms and lowering them, imagine the whole body relaxed with smooth flow of *Qi* and blood.

3. 两掌上托和下落时，意念调整呼吸，气息归元。

When lifting and lowering both palms, regulate your breathing and return *Qi* to its origin.

4. 起身时要借助手脚的撑力，保持平衡，动作要连贯、稳健。

When standing up, rely on the support of the hands and feet to maintain balance, and make sure the movements are smooth and steady.

三、功理功用
III. Functions and Effects

本式动作可放松肢体，平和气息，愉悦心情，恢复常态。

This posture can relax your body, calm the breath, and restore normal state with a pleasant mood.

四、适宜症状
IV. Indications

可缓解内心焦虑，精神紧张等症状。

It can alleviate symptoms such as inner anxiety and mental stress.

十二段锦的呼吸要求

Breathing Requirements

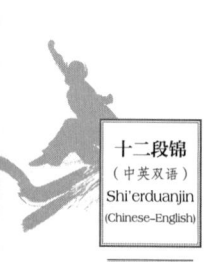

十二段锦对呼吸的总体要求是，在初学阶段采取自然呼吸。动作熟练后，配合不同的呼吸要求进行练习。"冥心握固""叩齿鸣鼓""摇身晃海"等式均采用自然呼吸，不改变自己正常的呼吸方式，顺其自然地呼吸，不加任何意念控制。"温煦脐轮"一式采用顺腹式呼吸，吸气时腹部隆起，呼气时腹部内收。"微撼天柱""掌抱昆仑""摇转辘轳""托天按顶""俯身攀足""前抚脘腹""鼓漱吞津"等式均采用逆腹式呼吸并配合提肛呼吸，吸气时腹部内收，有意识地收提肛门及会阴部肌肉，呼气时腹部隆起，放松肛门及会阴部肌肉。"背摩精门"一式中的两掌合拢做拧转翻落动作及收势中的两手握拳胸前交叉，均采用闭气的方式，在吸气结束后屏住呼吸，闭气时间长短根据动作的要求和个人状况决定。

The overall requirement for breathing in Shi'erduanjin is to adopt natural breathing during the initial learning stage. After becoming proficient in the movements, practice with different kinds of breathing. The postures of "Calm Mind and Clench Hands", "Click Teeth and Sound Drums", and "Rotate Upper Body" all use natural breathing, without changing one's normal breathing pattern and without any intentional control. The posture of "Warm Navel Ring" uses abdominal breathing, with the abdomen rising when inhaling and contracting when exhaling. The postures of "Slightly Shake Heavenly Column", "Hold *Kunlun* in Hands", "Rotate Arms like Windlass", "Hold Up Heaven and Press Crown", "Bend to Touch Feet", "Caress Upper and Lower Abdomen", and "Gargle and Swallow" all use reverse abdominal breathing, combined with anal sphincter breathing.

When inhaling, contract the abdomen, consciously lifting the anus and perineum muscles. When exhaling, arch the abdomen, relaxing the anus and perineum muscles. When twisting and lowering the clasped hands in the posture of "Massage Essence Gates" and crossing the wrists in front of the chest in the posture of "Closing", hold your breath. After completing the inhalation, hold breath for a while, which varies according to the requirement of the movement and the individual's condition.

学习建议
Learning Tips

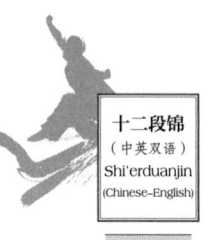

1. 清楚动作的路线和节点。

Know clearly the route and transitional movements.

2. 感悟动作的要求、要领和呼吸方法。

Comprehend the requirements, essentials and breathing methods of every movement.

3. 了解和掌握动作所涉及的脏腑经络和穴位。

Understand and master the internal organs, meridians and acupoints involved in every movement.

4. 松贯始终，一点儿紧一片松，才能够更好地导引气血，使全身经脉畅通。

Keep your body relaxed throughout the practice. "Part tenseness with general relaxation" can better guide the flow of *Qi* and blood and improve the circulation of *Qi* in meridians.

5. 练功之前做好腰腿部准备活动，初练时宜采用自然盘坐势。

Before practicing, warm up the waist and legs. It is recommended to start with a natural cross-legged sitting position.

6. 盘坐时如腰腿出现疼痛、麻木等现象，应及时调整，不可忍耐强行。

If there is any pain or numbness in the lower back or legs while sitting in the cross-legged position, adjust it promptly. Do not force yourself to bear it.